THERE IS AN ALTERNATIVE TO ASPIRIN!

Whether you suffer from osteoarthritis, rheumatoid arthritis, gout—or any other type of arthritis, the facts, advice and techniques in NATURAL RELIEF FOR ARTHRITIS can change your life. You'll find:

- How the elimination of fat, sugar and salt from your diet can help free you from pain
- Why B vitamins work as treatment
- How water provides amazing relief from arthritis
- Stretching exercises for stronger, more flexible joints

And much more!

———————————

"A wide-ranging source of information and help . . . a conscientious presentation of orthodox and alternative possibilities."

—*Kirkus Reviews*

"Virtually the only arthritis book available that addresses such a diversity of conventional and unconventional therapies."

—*Library Journal*

Natural
Relief For
ARTHRITIS

Carol Keough

and the editors of
PREVENTION® magazine

PUBLISHED BY POCKET BOOKS NEW YORK

POCKET BOOKS, a division of Simon & Schuster, Inc.
1230 Avenue of the Americas, New York, N.Y. 10020

Published by arrangement with Rodale Press, Inc.
Library of Congress Catalog Card Number: 82-23111

ISBN: 0-671-60411-2

First Pocket Books printing November, 1986

10 9 8 7 6 5 4 3 2 1

POCKET and colophon are registered
trademarks of Simon & Schuster, Inc.

Printed in the U.S.A.

Contents

List of Tables

List of Boxes

Acknowledgments

My sincere thanks go to the many health professionals who most graciously shared their information and expertise, especially: Joseph Lee Hollander, M.D.; Roger Hollister, M.D.; Steve Pickert, M.D.; Gary Emery, Ph.D.; Ray Wunderlich, M.D.; Ann Fettner; William Kaufman, M.D., Ph.D.; Lawrence Power, M.D.; Nathan Pritikin; Marshall Mandell, M.D.; James Braly, M.D.; and Norman F. Childers, Ph.D.

I'm also grateful for the generous help and advice offered to me by those with arthritis—Blanche Voss, Janet Wheeler, Betty Ford, Mitchel Greene, Sean Barrett, Susan Laird, and Tom Mealey. Thanks, too, for the contributions of my fellow editors, Eileen Mazer, Sharon Faelten, Stefan Bechtel, and Emrika Padus.

I especially want to acknowledge the contribution of Sue Ann Gursky, who inventively researched for this book, patiently compiled charts and tables, and carefully verified the facts that were stated. And thanks, too, to Bill Gottlieb, for his encouragement and gentle editing. And to Diana Gottshall and Susan Lagler for typing a long and sometimes scribbled manuscript.

Finally, special thanks to Anna Kopsay, my mother, who has arthritis and was the inspiration for this book.

Part 1

WHAT'S A NICE PERSON LIKE YOU DOING WITH A JOINT LIKE THIS?

1

THE NATURE OF
ARTHRITIS

Sparkles from the mirrored globe swim along the walls. The band thumps, "Celebrate, good times, come ON." Bodies wiggle and sweat on the dance floor. Elizabeth, a stunning blonde in a blue silk dress, beams her perfect smile at her gyrating friends. She sits alone at the table, carefully keeping her hands on her lap where no one can see her twisted fingers. She keeps her feet, in their sturdy black oxfords, hidden under the table.

Elizabeth is 25, and has rheumatoid arthritis.

* * *

Carl Widmer is a very successful businessman. Most people think his success results from his sincerity and friendliness. He's a really nice guy.

Twice a year, Carl attends an industry convention where he wines and dines clients and potential clients. He begins each day with a bacon 'n' eggs business breakfast, punctuates it with a meat 'n' potatoes business lunch, and culminates it with a gourmet dinner and lots of drinks. He follows this routine for five days straight.

At the end of the week, two things always result. Carl gets lots of orders and a case of the gout.

* * *

The kids on the block call her Mrs. M. She's a fixture in her little neighborhood in New York City. She is the feeder of stray cats, the cookie baker, the birthday card sender, and the lady who can tell you how to cure a sick houseplant.

Mrs. M., who is in her mid-seventies, always felt pretty well. She's had aching and stiff knees for more than ten years. She has trouble climbing stairs and getting out of deep chairs, but generally she's maintained all her activities. And her good humor.

But lately, Mrs. M. hasn't been herself. Her hair, normally shining white and attractively curled, is dull and limp. Mrs. M. can't raise her arms to properly wash and set it. She has trouble getting dressed in the morning, so sometimes she stays in her bathrobe all day. She looks in the mirror and sighs, "Getting old."

She's depressed about her appearance and tired of her aches and pains. She doesn't sit outdoors so often anymore, and the stray cats have moved on, looking for another soft touch.

Mrs. M. has osteoarthritis.

* * *

Frankie is a cute kid of 12. He's involved in Scouts and Little League baseball, and does pretty well in school. Lately, he's had a fever and a rash. The pains in his wrists, knuckles, and knees may not be just growing pains after all. His doctor thinks he might have juvenile arthritis—but it's a tough disease to diagnose. Frankie just wants to get back on the team before the season ends. He wishes everyone would stop poking at him.

* * *

Arthritis is not quite as common as the common cold. But it comes close. Surveys show that 31.6 *million* people, or 14 percent of the population, suffer some form of arthritis serious enough to require medical treatment. Each year, arthritis snares 1 million new victims. So, if you have arthritis, you've got plenty of company.

Because of arthritis, 26.6 million work days are lost each year. That is the equivalent of an astounding 72,877 years of labor down the drain. And that figure represents just the tally of those days missed from regular paying jobs, and doesn't include the uncounted millions of sick days lost by house-wives, students, retirees, and part-time workers.

We can recount lots of statistics about this disease, but, in many ways, arthritis itself remains a mystery. It exists in more than 100 guises, ranging from the older person's creaking knees to the jock's tennis elbow and the epicure's torturous gouty toe. The common element of all these variations is pain in the joints or spine. Some people with arthritis may simply have a single, painful joint that yields to a month of drug therapy, nutritional therapy, or no therapy at all. For others, arthritis can be a vicious, agonizing condition that inexorably spreads through every joint in the body. It can be caused by bacteria, by a virus, or by a disruption in body chemistry.

The two most common forms of arthritis are osteo-arthritis and rheumatoid arthritis. These are real mysteries because no one knows what causes them. And no one can predict how bad the disease will be in any given person. For example, osteoarthritis—the wear-and-tear joint disease that almost everyone will get if they live long enough—can remain just a mere nuisance for some people, but can cripple others. Rheumatoid arthritis is equally puzzling. It follows such an erratic course that it has been described as a river that never flows the same way twice. It can appear, lie low for a number of years, then flare like a bonfire that is hot and all-consuming. Or it can just go away all by itself, and never return. Fortunately, in 10 to 20 percent of cases, it does just that.

Arthritis, in other words, can be a harsh, unpredictable, and frustrating enemy. But wait! Despite all these unknowns, the disease can be outwitted. While medicine has not found a sure cure, it has found effective treatments that offer relief. Home treatment can make the difference between being a person who happens to have arthritis and an arthritic—that is, a person who is defined by his disease. But if you make a deep personal commitment to fighting the disease, it will be held at bay. That intangible x-factor—your own attitude—can make the whole difference between whether your arthritis is a minor pain or a major disability.

So, if you're willing to consign your bones to that old rocking chair, that's just where you'll stay for the rest of your days. But if you want to remain in the thick of things, vital and full of life, then start today to plot your strategy. Your weapons against arthritis are rest, exercise, medical treatment, good nutrition, and a strong will to keep going.

Who Gets Arthritis?

The answer, unfortunately, is that almost everybody gets it, if they live long enough. Many people believe that only those who live in a cold, damp climate usually get the disease. However, this does not seem to be the case. A few years ago, a medical research team from the National Institute of Arthritis, Metabolism, and Digestive Diseases set out to determine whether rheumatoid arthritis is more common in a cold, damp climate than in a warm, dry one. They studied two Indian tribes, reasoning that each group was fairly stationary and therefore lived their entire lives in the same sort of environment. They compared the Blackfeet, who dwell in the wintery climate of Montana, with the Pima, who live in the hot, dry Southwest. What the researchers found was surprising. The desert Indians actually had a few *more* cases of arthritis than their Montana counterparts.

It doesn't seem to matter whether you live in sunny California or wet and windy Syracuse, New York. You're equally likely to develop the disease in either place. What does seem to matter is your sex. Women tend to suffer more from the common forms of arthritis, but men are the usual victims of the more unusual types.

For example, rheumatoid arthritis strikes three times more women than men. But it seems to single out just certain *kinds* of women. A U.S. National Health Survey revealed that it skips over most unmarried women and women over 45. As for men, the same survey showed that it generally does not strike widowed men. Moreover, the more managerial a man's job, the less prone he is to getting rheumatoid arthritis.

Because osteoarthritis is the most common form of the disease, there are plenty of both men and women affected by it. The disease is rare in children and young adults, but begins to twinge the joints of those in their middle years. One type of arthritis, however, does single out just women. Usually striking them after their fortieth birthday, it forms bony little knobs at the end joints of the fingers. These knobs, called Heberden's nodes, tend to run in families. While they can be painful, they often don't limit the use of the fingers.

While women seem to take the brunt of these two major forms of arthritis, gout is a man's disease. It strikes between the ages of 30 and 50. It, too, seems to run in families, but diet also plays a major role.

Another common form of arthritis affects the spine. The tongue-twister name of this inflammatory disease is ankylosing spondylitis, and it hits ten times as many men as women. It's a young man's disease, striking between the ages of 20 and 30.

Also included in the grab bag of diseases called "arthritis" are problems of sore, stiff joints that really aren't caused by arthritis at all. These include traumatic arthritis (where a joint has been injured by a blow or strain), bursitis, back strain, joint infections that result from venereal disease, a staph infection, or even a virus carried by ticks. Stress and your general mental and emotional state also come into play when arthritis flares up.

Age is another major factor in arthritis of all kinds. According to a 1976 health survey, there are only 7.1 million people under the age of 45 who have arthritis. But that figure jumps dramatically to 43.3 million arthritics between the ages of 45 and 64. Another 21.8 million people over 65 also suffer from arthritis. In fact, studies show that about 97 percent of all people over 60 have arthritis severely enough for it to show up on X rays. Seeing the enormity of these figures, you certainly can realize why arthritis is called the nation's number one crippling disease.

What Causes Arthritis?

As you can see, men are susceptible to some forms of arthritis while women are prone to others. However, man or woman, the older you get, the more likely you are to develop some form of the illness. But there are no hard and fast rules for this tricky disease. Some young people do get it while many older people do not. Some cases are severe enough to cripple, while others are nothing more than nuisance twinges. Arthritis has left medical science searching for explanations. Most doctors can only agree that if a joint functions perfectly, it isn't likely to degenerate into osteoarthritis. But if a joint has taken a lot of punishment over the years—because you are a feisty competitor on the playing field, or because you're simply overweight—parts of the joints may begin to wear away. Also, if the joint was less than perfect to begin with—if it had a hidden defect—that, too, could result in osteoarthritis.

The causes of other forms of arthritis are still unknown. One medical theory holds that our body's own immune system somehow goes haywire. Instead of fighting foreign matter like germs, it attacks parts of our own bodies, resulting in injury to cartilage, bone, muscles, and other tissues. Another theory holds that this Kamikaze defense system is set in motion by a virus-type organism that hides in the body, perhaps hibernating for years. Suddenly, something, maybe illness or emotional stress, triggers it into action. The result is inflammation of the joints.

It's disappointing that medical science does not know more about the disease. It is one of the oldest known to humanity. If you were to visit the Museum of Natural History at the University of Kansas, you could view the skeleton of a reptile estimated to be 100 million years old, and see the effects of multiple arthritis. Chronic arthritis of the spine is known to have plagued prehistoric man (and woman). Egyptian mummies show its effects. And the ancient Romans built luxurious baths throughout their empire to help ease the pains in their joints. This most common form of the disease—osteoarthritis—has been with humankind since the day we first stood up.

Arthritis: Art and History

But scientists don't have a clear idea of when the other common form—rheumatoid arthritis—became so prevalent. Some historians believe the increase in people suffering with this ailment coincided with the Industrial Revolution, and might in some mysterious way be linked to it. However, a recent study done by four doctors with an eye for art reports that rheumatoid arthritis may have existed at least two centuries before the Industrial Revolution. These doctors, three from Belgium and one from Philadelphia, reviewed the paintings of Peter Paul Rubens, who lived from 1577 to 1640, a time considerably before the beginnings of modern industry. The doctors knew that Rubens was a realistic painter, but that, to please his patrons, he often left out their more unattractive features. Consequently, the people portrayed in his beautiful paintings appeared without warts, potbellies, or pimples. You can imagine how fascinated the doctors were, therefore, to find images of knobby fingers, swollen wrists and knees, dilated veins, and other clearly recognizable signs of what had to be rheumatoid arthritis.

To be certain they could push the date of the start of rheumatoid arthritis back two centuries, the doctors submitted the paintings to independent review by artists, rheumatologists, and doctors who were specialists in other areas of medicine. They all generally agreed that, yes indeed, it *was* rheumatoid arthritis depicted in those seventeenth-century paintings.

But why? Dr. George Ehrlich, the American of the investigative quartet, says that the portrayal of such deformities could actually be a form of signature. He notes that the swollen joints and knobby fingers in the artworks become progressively worse over the years that Rubens painted them. But they are not shown on only one subject—whose arthritis was getting more and more severe. Instead, they are shown on a variety of different subjects, ranging from Saint Anne in the painting *The Holy Family with Saint Anne* to the master, himself.

The doctors' study, printed in the *Journal of the American Medical Association,* concludes, "The accurately detailed progression in his work suggests it was a painter and not a model in whom the disease was so carefully portrayed."

Of course, arthritis is not an affliction that targets just painters. Christopher Columbus, Cardinal Richelieu, Mary, Queen of Scots, President James Madison, Horace the poet, Julius Caesar, Augustus Caesar, John Calvin, and Pope Pius II all made their way into the pages of history despite having the disease. Many more of the famous also must have suffered with the disease, but for their own reasons, concealed it from the public.

Today, things have changed and a number of well-known people have "gone public" about their arthritis, hoping to set a good example of what is possible in life, even a life limited by a disease with no known cure. Consequently, people with arthritis sometimes now turn up on television. For example, Dick Butkus, the former professional football player, has appeared on the "Tic Tac Dough" show, attempting to win money for the Arthritis Foundation. When host Wink Martindale asked Butkus if he keeps up his muscular physique by running, Butkus honestly answered that his bad knee keeps him from that particular exercise, but that the hours of therapy he spends to counter his arthritis keep him in shape.

Former First Lady Betty Ford also appears on television around the country, offering a message of hope. She says, "I'm Betty Ford, and like 30 million Americans I have arthritis. Arthritis means living with pain. Everyday activities we all take for granted become unbearable. But thanks to medical advances, I can now cope with my arthritis. You can find help, too."

Other well-known people coping daily include: the actors Elizabeth Taylor, Arthur Godfrey, Katharine Hepburn, James Garner, Buddy Ebsen, Ricardo Montalban, Raymond Massey, and John Carradine; newsman Eric Sevareid; orchestra conductor Eugene Ormandy; dancers Edward Villela and Martha Graham; athletes Joe Namath, Dick Butkus, Wes Unseld, and Bruce Furniss; surgeon Christiaan Barnard; and President Ronald Reagan.

If they can cope, so can you.

2

OSTEOARTHRITIS: WHEN JOINTS ARE WORN AND TORN

Like Rodney Dangerfield, people with osteoarthritis often feel "they don't get no respect." Your knees or back can ache like mad, but your friends just shrug and say, "What do you expect? You're getting old." And when you finally haul your sore body to the doctor, what does *he* say? "What do you expect? You're getting old."

Meanwhile, you're beginning to feel emotionally depressed because it hurts to do so many tasks you never had to think twice about doing before. Maybe you don't mind terribly that you're no longer in any condition to paint the siding on the house, but when you have to cancel a tennis match or a day on the golf course, it can get to you. And, as the disease progresses, you feel more pain in more joints. Eventually, some people get such bad osteoarthritis they view a flight of stairs as the equivalent of Mt. Everest. Squatting down to pet the dog can be a memorable event—because of the pain.

What exactly is this form of misery that has been visited on your joints? And what can you do about it?

What Is Osteoarthritis?

Osteoarthritis, the most common form of arthritis, is characterized by pain and stiffness in the joints. Usually, osteoarthritis is limited to only one or two parts of the body—the fingers, knees, hips, neck, or low back. Men tend to get it in their hips, while women generally get it in their hands. It tends to strike both sides of the body, so if you start out having pain in your right knee, soon you'll also have pain in the left. Generally, the joint on the dominant side of the body is affected first.

A survey of people with osteoarthritis showed that 75 percent had arthritis in their knees, 60 percent had it in their hands, 25 percent in their hips, and a small number had problems with their ankles and shoulders. Usually, osteoarthritis doesn't hit the elbows or wrists. About a third of the people surveyed also had trouble with osteoarthritis in the spine.

The disease usually surfaces suddenly, often around age 50. It seems that your occupation can have some effect on which joints it strikes. For example, studies show that coal miners get it in their knees, cotton workers get it in their hands, and pneumatic drill operators get it in their wrists. It seems that osteoarthritis affects a stressed joint first. In addition to stress created by the type of work you do, stress also includes carrying too heavy a burden. For that reason, overweight people frequently wind up with osteoarthritis in their knees. In addition, any joint that has been fractured is a prime candidate for osteoarthritis.

The disease usually makes its presence known to someone in his 50s, but X rays show the deterioration actually begins long before. Degenerative changes start as early as age 20, and by the time we reach our fortieth birthday, 90 percent of us have some arthritic changes in the joints that bear weight. After age 55, almost everyone has osteoarthritis to some degree. It's a disease that develops slowly, and quite literally sneaks up on you like a thief in the night.

Generally, people with osteoarthritis don't feel sick. That is, they don't have a fever or a loss of appetite. The disease is limited to the joints and—even in the worst possible cases—is never, ever fatal.

JUST ANOTHER DAY

Blanche Voss, 70, has a bad case of osteoarthritis. She's had the illness for the past 25 years, and it now dictates how she will spend her day.

"I never make early appointments," she explains. "In the morning, I'm just miserable. I take a pill as soon as I wake up. Then, four hours later, I take a second pill. By then I finally can move around.

"I'd like to do more, but I'm afraid to commit myself to a job or a group. I'd like to help out at the hospital. But the world starts early in the morning, and I'm just not in tune with it."

It's the world's loss, really. Blanche is a Phi Beta Kappa graduate of the University of Chicago, and has much to offer. But her arthritis limits her goals as well as her physical activities.

"I feel very depressed sometimes. Wouldn't you? To wake up *every* morning feeling horrible."

But Blanche gamely insists she leads a normal life. "I'm not a *cripple,* and I keep going," she says.

With osteoarthritis, the day has a lot of ups and downs. Typically, you wake up feeling stiff, and require 15 minutes to a half hour to "thaw." Generally, you feel some pain when you move the affected joint, but as the day progresses, it begins to feel better. Often, by early afternoon your condition has improved, but as the day wears on the pain begins to build again. By evening it reaches its peak.

Sometimes when the pain is not bad, you can attempt a fairly strenuous chore—like washing some windows or digging in the garden. But after unusually vigorous exercise, the sore joints will hurt even more than ever.

Stiffness, too, comes and goes during the day. You wake up stiff because your joints have not been exercised during the night. Once you get moving, the stiffness goes away. But if you settle down to read or watch television for an hour or so, it returns.

Yet another symptom is the cracking, grinding, or popping of arthritic joints. While this symptom is not serious—it doesn't cause pain or limit motion—it is often the most embarrassing aspect of having osteoarthritis. A good knee crack, after all, can be heard at a considerable distance and always seems its resounding loudest in church or at a party.

My friend Jan Wheeler was diagnosed as having osteoarthritis. In some ways, she is a perfect example of a textbook case. But there's one major difference—the disease hasn't bothered her a bit in the last two years. She's 55 now, and at 5 feet, 2 inches, and 105 pounds, she has the figure of a schoolgirl. She made a conscious effort all her life to keep that figure by exercising. She's a regular in local tennis tournaments and works out frequently at a gym.

"I've always been active," says Jan. "The day before I got the pain, I was doing some gardening that involved putting in railroad ties and circular cement slabs. Later that day, I was moving a box spring and mattress, and I just fell. I had to laugh at myself for acting like I'm still 23.

"The next morning I woke up with a pain that started at the back of my neck and went down my left arm and into my hand. Four of my fingers were numb, and I couldn't feel anything that I picked up. I couldn't even make myself a cup of tea."

Jan, who is a widow and lives alone, got very frightened. "I'm going to have to depend on someone to take care of me," she worried. In a very uncharacteristic move, Jan took the next three days off from work. "I stayed home in bed, trying to sleep and hoping the pain would be gone when I woke up. But it didn't go away."

Jan then began the rounds of doctors and hospitals. She started with an osteopath who, after taking blood tests and X rays, diagnosed her as having a very bad case of osteoarthritis that had reached the degenerative stage. "I went to him for ultrasound treatments, but they really didn't help me," she said.

Next, she went to a medical doctor, who gave her a complete physical, including X rays, blood tests, and even a rectal examination. "At first, he said he didn't think I had arthritis. But after the X rays came in, he said there was no doubt about it. He told me to take aspirin, maybe two, four times a day. I didn't like the idea of taking all that aspirin, because it always upsets my stomach."

Finally, Jan went to a chiropractor, who gave her ten adjustments to align her bones. "He also suggested that I supplement my diet with thiamine, alfalfa, calcium lactate, magnesium oxide, dolomite, lecithin, bone meal, zinc, beef liver extract, and the vitamins C, E, B_6, and B_{12}.

"You know what?" smiles Jan. "I've felt fine ever since, except for a tiny numb spot at the tip of my left pinky."

According to Jan, the worst part of her bout with arthritis was the fear. "The more worried I got, the more pain I had. I really think that tension and aggravation have a lot to do with the way you tolerate pain, or even how much pain you have. I also found out that rest and relaxation can make you feel much better."

As the years go by, a person with osteoarthritis will find that he or she has long periods of "normal" joint pain punctuated by attacks of acute pain. Once a joint is involved, it stays involved. Often, other joints are added over the years.

Types and Causes

There are two basic types of osteoarthritis: primary and secondary. Primary osteoarthritis just happens. It has no obvious cause. One morning you wake up with a stiff shoulder that hurts when you move it, and you can't think of a single thing you did the day before that could have caused the problem. Primary osteoarthritis includes Heberden's nodes and other age-related joint problems.

Secondary osteoarthritis doesn't just happen. It is caused by a clearly identifiable problem. For example, if a joint is injured in any way, it's likely to develop problems later. Other causes of secondary osteoarthritis include old fractures, infections inside the joint, tissue damage caused by diseases like diabetes or gout, overuse of drugs injected directly into the joint, or deposits of calcium in the cartilage.

There's much debate in medical literature about whether osteoarthritis should be considered an inflammatory disease. One group holds that the disease is limited to cartilage degeneration, with very little inflammation present, and therefore is not an inflammatory disease. If your doctor is among this group he may even call your illness *osteoarthrosis,* because the *itis* part of osteoarthritis implies inflammation.

Another group of doctors does consider osteoarthritis to be inflammatory. Joseph Lee Hollander, M.D., professor emeritus of medicine at the University of Pennsylvania School of Medicine and the "dean" of arthritis medicine in this country, says that even though inflammatory cells are *not* present in a sore joint, osteoarthritis has an inflammatory nature.

Following the strict definition of inflammation, he says we would have to regard a blister which develops on the heel after long walking in a poor-fitting shoe as noninflammatory because the fluid in the blister doesn't contain any inflammatory cells. "However," he says, "most of us feel that such a painful hot and tender swelling *is* inflammatory, even though engendered by friction rather than by infection or deposit of foreign material, so I regard the painful joints of osteoarthritis as inflammatory."

This group also notes that anti-inflammatory drugs often help relieve the joint pain of osteoarthritis.

Seeing the Doctor

If you've had a sore or stiff joint for a month or two, you ought to see a doctor. He'll manipulate the joints that hurt, feel for heat, prod for swelling, and listen for any grinding or popping noises. Before he makes his diagnosis, he also may require you to take some tests. Generally, these would include X rays, a Sedimentation Rate test, perhaps an examination of fluid taken from the sore joint, and possibly a Rheumatoid Factor test.

X RAYS

X rays are a common tool in diagnosing osteoarthritis. The X rays pass right through the joint tissue, but they do reveal the presence of bone spurs (osteophytes) that develop during the course of osteoarthritis. X rays will also show a narrowing of the space between the two bones that meet inside the joint. That narrowing indicates that the cartilage protecting the ends of the bone has begun to wear away.

Because X rays expose you to dangerous radiation, avoid them if possible. Often a doctor can tell just as much about a joint just by physically examining it.

SEDIMENTATION RATE TEST
OR "SED RATE"

This test is a "blood test." The doctor or laboratory technician will draw blood from you. It will be held in a test tube until the two main components of the blood—the solid cells and the liquid serum in which they float—separate into layers. The distance that the cells settle in one hour is the sedimentation rate. A high "sed rate" means inflammation is present. The higher the sed rate, the greater the inflammation. By taking this test periodically, a doctor can tell if the inflammation in a patient's joints is getting better or worse.

In cases of osteoarthritis, the sedimentation rate is usually normal. In cases of rheumatoid arthritis, the sedimentation rate is usually high. Thus, this test can help the doctor distinguish between the two types of arthritis.

JOINT FLUID TEST

A needle is inserted into the sore joint and a few drops of joint fluid (synovial fluid) are drawn out. This fluid can tell a lot about what is going on inside the joint. For example, in cases of osteoarthritis, the fluid is usually clear and sticky, but contains some debris from the cartilage that's wearing out inside the joint. If the problem inside the joint is not caused by the cartilage, but by an infection, the bacteria in the fluid can be cultured and identified. If the fluid contains crystals of uric acid, the problem in the joint is most likely caused by gout.

RHEUMATOID FACTOR TEST

This is a blood test that searches specifically for a rheumatoid factor circulating in the blood. This "factor" is something the body's immune system produces to fight off rheumatoid disease. Its presence in the blood means the patient probably has rheumatoid arthritis (RA), not osteoarthritis.

When the examination and all the tests have been completed, the doctor will be able to tell you with certainty whether you have osteoarthritis, or perhaps just a local injury to the joint, an infection, or some more serious form of the disease like RA or lupus erythematosus. You may be told to take aspirin, to exercise, and/or rest. The doctor may talk to you about joint degeneration, aging, problems with cartilage or joint membranes, inherited disorders, metabolic disorders, and more. Unless you know something about anatomy, the advice you get may seem conflicting and confusing.

IT'S TIME TO SEE YOUR DOCTOR, IF—

you have a combination of the following symptoms:

- a joint has been painful for more than five to six weeks
- it hurts when you move it
- it stiffens after a long rest
- it hurts most in the evening
- it makes a cracking or grinding sound when moving
- it is close to a bone that was broken
- it was injured in the past
- it is hot and swollen
- if one or both parents have osteoarthritis
- if you have small bumps at the end joints of one or more fingers.

Inside the Joint

To understand what's happening to you when you have osteoarthritis, it's important to visualize the structure of a joint. Bones come together inside a joint capsule, where the ends that meet are lubricated and cushioned so they can slide easily past each other to assume their new flexed or straightened position. The capsule itself is made of tough fibrous

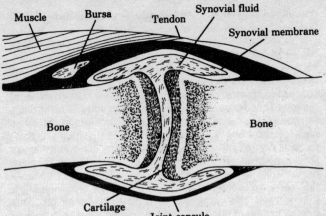

Muscle Bursa Tendon Synovial fluid

Synovial membrane

Bone Bone

Cartilage Joint capsule

Inside the joint capsule, the ends of the bones are protected and lubricated by the synovial membrane. The end of each bone is covered by a smooth layer of cartilage that allows the bones to slide easily past each other. Osteoarthritis is a disease that causes this cartilage to flake and wear away. In advanced cases, raw bone rubs against raw bone. Usually, spurs form at the ends of the bone. Called osteophytes, they are visible as "knobs" on arthritic joints.

tissue. Inside it is a membrane that surrounds the joint. It is called the synovial membrane, and provides the joint's lubricating fluid. Muscles taper down to become tendons and attach to the bone at the joint.

Let's visualize what happens, for example, when you bend your elbow. You begin by flexing your arm muscle, which pulls on the tendon, which moves the bone, which bends the joint. Voila! One bent elbow.

In some parts of the body, there are bursae—little pouches containing a gummy fluid—that provide extra lubrication for body tissues that have to move against each other.

At the heart of the joint are the two bones that meet and move. The tip of each bone is covered with a silky smooth layer of cartilage that not only provides a nonfriction surface that allows the bones to slide easily, but also absorbs shock. Osteoarthritis is a disease of that cartilage.

In the first stages of the disease, the swollen cartilage begins to flake as though it's been sandpapered. After a time, vertical cracks appear. These are deep and dangerous. Cartilage cells mass in colonies around these clefts, but don't succeed in repairing the tissue. At this point of degeneration, the joint is under considerable strain. The body, in an attempt to protect itself, lays down some extra calcium at the outer ends of the bone where the tendons or ligaments are attached. As a result of this extra calcium, little bony spurs form inside the joint. These are called osteophytes. They are most visible as the bony knobs—called Heberden's nodes—that show up at the end joints of the fingers. Occasionally, a jolt or twist can cause the osteophyte to break off. This unattached bit of bone is commonly called a joint mouse, and it moves about inside the joint space. Occasionally, a mouse will get caught between the two bones as they move, causing an excruciating pain.

As the cartilage degenerates and osteophytes form, the synovial membrane covering the joint also suffers. The blood vessels in the membrane become narrowed, reducing blood flow. This reduction creates two problems. As the joint is used, friction causes heat to build. But the blood flow is insufficient to dissipate the heat and carry it away. Secondly, when the joint is at rest, the synovial membrane stiffens, leading to a "gelling" inside that makes the joint difficult to move.

Ultimately, the combination of stiffness, cartilage degeneration, and bone formation can interfere with the joint's ability to function normally.

The mechanics of what's happening inside the joint are fairly easy to understand. What's difficult is finding out what *causes* normal, healthy cartilage to begin flaking and cracking until it wears away. Generally, medical science has always believed it was simply the result of wear and tear. As the years add up, so do all the little shocks, bumps, and glitches that happen to a joint. This kind of daily grind can wear out rugs, shoes, tires, and furniture, so it seems logical that it should have the same effect on your joints. Therefore, it's often said that osteoarthritis is the inevitable result of aging, and will happen to anyone who lives long enough.

· Exciting Medical Breakthrough

So it seems we have a disease we cannot prevent and cannot cure. However, some new discoveries in medicine may put this bleak view to rest. Doctors are beginning to think that just because a disease *comes* with age does not always mean it is *caused* by age. First of all, we know that certain other forms of arthritis, like gout, are hereditary. We also know that some variations of osteoarthritis itself, like Heberden's nodes, also are hereditary. The implication is that there may be some inherited weakness that allows for the disintegration of cartilage.

Doctors at St. Bartholomew's Hospital and Medical College in London believe they may have found this inherited disorder, while doctors on this side of the Atlantic have found evidence that cartilage *can* sometimes repair itself.

In England, researchers were looking for a cause for another kind of arthritis—one called pseudogout—when they stumbled upon what may be a major discovery. They had drawn fluid from the joints of arthritis patients and were examining it for traces of a mineral known to cause pseudogout. Instead, they discovered something else in the fluid—crystals so tiny they can be seen only under an electron microscope. These crystals are made of a mineral called hydroxyapatite, which is the very same mineral that makes bones and teeth rigid. Dr. Derek A. Willoughby, director of research, rheumatology, and pathology at the hospital, had his research team investigate these crystals further. Joint fluid and tissue samples were supplied by ten collaborating European medical centers. The team examined the fluid from 100 patients with osteoarthritis. An astounding 74 of them had these hydroxyapatite crystals in their joint fluid.

Imagine throwing a handful of sand into your sneakers and running the Boston Marathon. Picture the size of the blisters you'd get, the amount of inflammation and the pain! That's the kind of damage these crystals can do to a joint. According to Dr. Willoughby, they roughen up the smooth cartilage and reduce its ability to cushion stress. As the crystals travel through the joint space they cause inflammation, tenderness, and swelling—all the standard symptoms of osteoarthritis.

To be positive it was the *crystals* causing the damage and not some other, unknown factor, the research team injected a tiny number of them into their own joints. Sure enough, the injected joints became sore, just as though the researchers had osteoarthritis. The degree of inflammation increased with the quantity and size of the crystals.

Further research showed that these crystals do not seem to come from the bones, even though the mineral is an essential part of bone formation. Instead, the researchers believe they are the result of an inherited disorder that throws off the body's ability to maintain a stable balance of calcium.

In this aspect, osteoarthritis may be considered similar to gout, which is also caused by an inherited disorder. In gout, excess uric acid in the body forms into crystals that inflame joints. In recent years, medicines have been developed to control both the frequency of gout attacks and their severity. The researchers at St. Bartholomew's Hospital are very hopeful that a new drug can be developed to control osteoarthritis in the same way—by preventing the formation of the crystals in the first place.

And so, the long-held view that osteoarthritis is simply part of growing old—an infirmity that we just have to grin and bear—is being reconsidered by modern medicine.

Another long-held view of osteoarthritis is also being held up to close scrutiny. Medicine has always believed that cartilage cannot repair itself, at least, not repair itself efficiently enough to make any substantial improvement after it has been damaged. Cartilage is unlike skin, which will grow back over a scraped knee, or bone that knits and becomes sturdy again. If cartilage is scuffed up, it not only stays scuffed but usually gets worse. So they believed.

Leon Sokoloff, M.D., says he's found a number of reasons to examine the unqualified validity of this concept. He reports evidence that cartilage sometimes *does* repair itself. Because of that process, it may be possible to slow down the progress of the disease, so that it never reaches its worst stages. He also thinks it may even be possible for the disease to reverse itself, so the joints become better with time rather than worse.

He bases his opinion on some studies made on patients who had undergone surgery for osteoarthritis. Where an artificial hip had been installed, and dead tissue removed, researchers found new cartilage growing on the bone that was protected by the metal device. While the new layer of cartilage was less than perfect, it did show that cartilage has the capability to repair itself. They concluded that it was the protection provided by the metal implant that made the process possible.

Dr. Sokoloff also reports that, after another kind of operation where bone had been cut to relieve mechanical stress on osteoarthritic hips, the damaged cartilage improved. Dr. Sokoloff says the major conclusion he can draw from these observations is that osteoarthritis may not be caused simply by the inability of cartilage to repair itself. Rather, the real crux of the problem may be that there are factors that keep the cartilage from repairing itself.

What does this development mean for people who are now suffering with osteoarthritis? Dr. Sokoloff says, "This carries with it a certain optimism for ultimate development of methods for retarding if not reversing the development of osteoarthritis."

Translation: There may be a cure in the future.

* * *

These encouraging findings mean osteoarthritis may not be Everyman's future. If you develop the disease, it may be possible to control it so that cartilage does not become damaged. If you've had the disease for some time, and the cartilage is already damaged, there soon may be a way to stimulate growth of new cartilage.

In the meantime, the way you *feel* about having osteoarthritis can have a major impact on your daily life. You can simply withdraw, as Blanche Voss has. Or, you can struggle to keep going. Visit relatives, keep appointments, make dates with friends. Wring some measure of satisfaction and joy from life—even life with osteoarthritis.

3

RHEUMATOID ARTHRITIS, THE WHOLE-BODY ILLNESS

The difference between rheumatoid arthritis (RA) and all other forms is so great they should not even share the same name. While most types of arthritis settle into a joint or the backbone to make it ache, RA is a disease of the whole body. A *systemic illness,* the doctors call it. With it come all the symptoms of a serious sickness—fever, chills, loss of appetite and body weight, sweating, morning stiffness, fatigue, and malaise.

The person with RA feels like he has a chronic infection, a virus, or the flu. But along with all these symptoms, he or she also suffers with hot, swollen, sore joints. The flu-like part of the disease can attack the muscles and skin; inflame the membranes that surround the heart and lungs; attack the lymph nodes, the whites of the eyes, and the small arteries; enlarge the spleen; and cause anemia.

When RA flares, it is as dangerous as any other major illness. It has the potential to cripple and even cause death.

While it's *possible* for RA to do all that harm, it rarely does. Fortunately, 20 percent of all people who get the disease simply recover completely. The majority of those with RA suffer occasional flare-ups and some joint pain, but generally have learned to live with a cyclical pattern of wellness and illness. These are the lucky folks who sought out an early diagnosis and got the inflammation under control before it could do a great deal of harm. Another 20 percent of those with RA can suffer permanent joint damage from the disease. Yet, everyone who has RA, even those with a resultant disability, find the disease easier to bear as time goes on, because it burns itself out.

The term rheumatoid arthritis (RA) often encompasses a small group of additional arthritic diseases that share a common feature—the inflammation of the synovial membrane. This group includes RA itself (sometimes called synovitis), juvenile rheumatoid arthritis, systemic lupus erythematosus, and psoriatic arthritis. Each of these illnesses will be discussed separately and in detail.

As we described in the previous chapter, the joint capsule is lined with the synovial membrane, whose function it is to lubricate the innards of the joint. In synovitis, the membrane becomes inflamed. It swells and begins to thicken. In severe cases, instead of looking like a swatch of satin, it looks more like a patch of shag rug. The joint becomes hot from increased blood flow, and swollen from the mobilized army of cells rushing to the joint to fight the inflammation.

Sometimes these inflammatory cells release an enzyme into the joint capsule. The enzyme was originally intended to fight foreign bodies like bacteria or viruses. However, if enough of the enzyme is released into the joint capsule for any length of time, it actually can digest the cartilage and bones inside the joint.

Although RA, juvenile rheumatoid arthritis, lupus, and psoriatic arthritis all share the common problem of synovitis, each also comes with its own set of additional symptoms, problems, and treatments. And each seems to favor a different segment of the population. Let's consider them one at a time.

Rheumatoid Arthritis

RA is a disease of the young. It generally affects those between 25 and 50, but can strike at any age. There are 6.5 million people in the United States today with RA, and three-quarters of them are women. No one knows why women are prone to this form of arthritis. Doctors have noted that the

○ Rheumatoid arthritis
● Osteoarthritis

Notice that osteoarthritis settles into the outmost joints of the hand, while rheumatoid arthritis strikes the lower joints and the wrist.

disease seems to diminish and even disappear during pregnancy, only to resurface after delivery. They, therefore, speculate that hormones may play a role in the disease, but they really don't know for sure.

RA usually strikes suddenly, beginning with a suspicious pain in one of the small joints. It usually hits the wrists and knuckles, but also is common in the knees or the joints that comprise the ball of the foot. If RA gravitates to the fingers it usually settles in the knuckles at the base of the finger, or sometimes in the middle knuckle, unlike osteoarthritis, which favors the end joint of the finger.

In addition to the limbs, RA can also affect the spine. In fact, 40 percent of all RA patients develop some arthritis in the upper spine, the section between the shoulder blades and the base of the skull. Usually, you feel pain when you move your neck. The pain can be so severe that it radiates to the forehead in blinding flashes. At times, it may not be possible to tilt your head backwards. If you try, pain and tingling shoot down the arms.

Betty Ford, wife of the former President, was stricken

with a similar form of arthritis at a time that was crucial in her husband's political life. In her book, *The Times of My Life*, she writes:

> In 1964, after the Goldwater-Miller convention, Jerry and I had made plans to spend some vacation time with all four children. The month was August, and we'd rented a cottage at Bethany Beach in Delaware for a couple of weeks.
>
> Two days before we were supposed to leave, I woke in the night with a terrible pain in my neck. The pain was shooting down my left arm, and that scared me. I couldn't sleep. I didn't want to disturb Jerry, so I went downstairs, and he found me there on the couch the next morning. He drove me over to National Orthopedic Hospital, and they put me to bed and into traction.
>
> I urged Jerry to go on, take the kids to the beach. He stayed away a week, then left the children with the mother of one of Mike's friends and came back to see how I was doing.
>
> I was doing lousy. They had me strung up to various devices and they were giving me gold shots. My problem had been diagnosed as a pinched nerve.
>
> How had I got it? Nobody knew. I blamed it on my having reached across a four-foot-wide counter in my kitchen to try to raise a window, but there's no way of proving that. The first time the hospital attendants took me for therapy, I cried from the pain. I couldn't lie down as they wanted me to and they had to work on my back while I sat on a chair and leaned forward across the treatment table.
>
> When I came home from the hospital, I was still holding my left arm across my chest, and I was all crouched over; I could have played the hunchback of Notre Dame.
>
> Jerry had a traction setup installed at home, and I spent another couple of weeks in bed.
>
> The day I got up, I glanced at myself in the full-length mirror in our bedroom, and I thought, My

lord, here I am, forty-six, and I look like an old woman of ninety. A crippled old woman.

I made up my mind I wasn't going to go on that way.

I started working on exercises to get myself back in an upright position, and to relax my arm, so it would hang by my side again and I wouldn't have to support it.

I continued my therapy, going to the National Orthopedic Hospital at least three times a week for hot packs and massage that loosened my muscles. I got so I could drive a car again, do the shopping, take over more of my duties as wife and mother. But, from that time to this, I've never been really free of the problem because I developed arthritis, and the combination of pinched nerve and spinal arthritis is really unpleasant. You don't have your arm in a sling, or your leg in a cast, you're not on crutches, and you try to appear as normal as possible, but you can't always fool people. A friend takes you by the hand, says "How do you feel?" and you say, "Fine, I'm fine," but the friend can see by your eyes that you're hurting.

In 1964 I was hurting, but I couldn't let that be the end of the line for me. I had a long way to go, four strapping children only half raised, a great responsibility.

Excerpted from The Times of My Life *by Betty Ford. Copyright © 1978 by Betty Ford. Reprinted by permission of Harper and Row, Publishers, Inc.*

When you have RA, you settle into a pattern with the disease. You live with it. While you never can consider it a friend, it is a predictable enemy. You know that if an attack comes on, it will strike suddenly and hard. Not only will the joints become very painful, hot and swollen, but, because of its systemic nature, you'll feel sick all over. Nobody will have to tell you to take your medicine and go to bed. You'll welcome them.

When joints are involved, they're usually the same on

both sides of the body. During an attack, severe inflammation can erode the joint. The damage is irreversible. But the disease permanently damages *only* the joints, not the eyes, arteries, and body organs that also can become inflamed.

In addition to pain and general malaise, many folks with RA also develop disfiguring nodules that form under the skin. They range in size from a small pea to a pearl onion, and signal the inflammation of a blood vessel. Usually, they pop out just below the elbow, or over some other bony outcropping. Sometimes they form over a bursa or tendon.

They're unattractive, but not permanent. They come and go. The only real hazard they pose is if they open and become infected. But nodules rarely open, unless they have formed in a spot that's under a lot of stress or subject to friction. Generally, this problem is limited to those lumps that develop on or near the ankles, which may swell frequently and put a lot of pressure on the nodules.

Generally, RA follows three basic patterns. One is called *monocyclic rheumatoid arthritis,* which lasts a few months, then goes away. Another is called *polycyclic rheumatoid arthritis,* which causes a series of attacks, but leaves you feeling well between bouts. The third is *chronic rheumatoid arthritis,* which is the kind most people with RA have.

In all cases, the disease becomes less aggressive as the years go by. You feel less tired and stiff. The synovial membrane becomes less inflamed, and no new joints become involved. And, all in all, only one person in six develops any crippling or deformities from his or her experience with RA.

The million dollar question is: what *causes* RA? It's been around at least since Shakespeare's time. It has afflicted uncounted millions all over the world. It's been studied by some of the world's finest medical minds, examined with the latest techniques using atomic age equipment, and what has been found?

No answers. Yet. But some clues, leads, hidden trails into unexplored areas of immunology, bacteriology, and heredity. Before we enter that jungle of biochemistry, let's make clear what doesn't cause RA. Despite the prevalence of the belief, it's not true that weather causes it. The correlation between weather and arthritis goes way back. In *A Midsummer Night's Dream,* Shakespeare wrote:

Therefore the moon, the governess of floods,
Pale in her anger, washes all the air,
That rheumatic diseases do abound:
And through this distemperature we see
The seasons alter: hoary-headed frosts
Fall in the fresh lap of the crimson rose.

Rain, cold, and a raw climate have wrongly been blamed for causing RA.

However, it *is* true that people with RA often can predict when the weather will turn foul.

Joseph Lee Hollander, M.D., one of the pioneers of rheumatology, once built a special chamber where all factors of the weather could be controlled. It was called the Climatron, and in it you could regulate the temperature, humidity, barometric pressure, air flow, and even the positive and negative ions in the air. People with RA were placed in the chamber, which was built at the Rehabilitation Center of the University of Pennsylvania Hospital in Philadelphia. It was found they felt more pain when the humidity went up and barometric pressure dropped—the same conditions that exist prior to a storm. In fact, 73 percent of all those who participated in the experiment had a worsening of their symptoms under these conditions.

Dr. Hollander built the Climatron as a result of his experiences during World War II, when he was stationed at Ashburn General Hospital in North Texas, where he took care of 65 soldiers who had arthritis.

"It was funny," he explains. "Every day I'd make my rounds and everyone would be okay. But every once in a while, there'd be a day when there were a lot more complaints. Now, it usually was sunny outside, with a cloudless sky. But the *next* day we'd get hit with a Blue Northern. This happened repeatedly. And I figured there must be something to this old wives' tale.

"What happens is that the diseased tissue cannot react to changing atmospheric conditions as quickly and as well as healthy tissue. A lot of people think they'll get better if they move to someplace like Arizona, but they won't. They might experience less pain because there are fewer weather changes in Arizona. But even if you could find the ideal climate and live there forever, you'd still have arthritis."

No, nothing so simple as the weather can explain so complex a disease as RA. The medical community has put forth several theories, and they run the gamut, including as possible causes everything from amoebae living in the bowel, and psychological disorders, to the body's own immune system run amok.

THE BODY ATTACKS ITSELF

The theory that seems most likely is that RA results from some malfunction in the immune system. Briefly, here's how it goes.

When the immune system is working properly, it produces cells that defend the body against matter that is foreign to the body, like germs or viruses. The body has two kinds of immunity. The first is called innate immunity, where your body instantly recognizes foreign matter and destroys it. The second is called adaptive immunity, where your body *learns* to recognize dangerous foreign matter. Vaccination, for example, brings about adaptive immunity. The adaptive system can recognize what is you and what is *not* you. Therefore, it doesn't send out an army of defender cells to attack and destroy your own tissue.

But, if your immune system malfunctions, that hoard of defender cells can turn traitor, and march on you. These cells are filled with a digestive enzyme. They surround and engulf what they believe is foreign matter, and simply digest it until it is totally destroyed. When this bizarre chain of events occurs, you are said to have an autoimmune disease.

Rheumatic fever, that kissin' cousin of RA, is an autoimmune disease. And so is lupus, which is one form of RA.

What would possibly make the very system designed to fight off disease suddenly *cause* a disease? Some believe it may be a hereditary defect. We pass our traits along through chromosomes and genes. These hold the key, for example, to whether we will have brown eyes or blue, be tall or short, and—maybe—be arthritic or not.

Researchers have examined the chromosomes of people with RA. They found a defect in the sixth set, the set that controls the development of the body's immune system, in 65 percent of those folks. But it's almost *never* found in people who don't have arthritis.

Another possible cause of immune malfunction is a virus. There is some evidence that RA may begin when a virus infection settles into a joint and causes an inflammation. Some doctors believe that if a virus penetrates into tissue cells, the body's defenses may fail to recognize the difference between the virus and the person's own tissue.

Scientists at a medical center in California found that people who have had a certain kind of virus—called Epstein-Barr virus—fought it off with a particular type of immune response. That same immune response is found in people who have RA. And so, doctors theorize that perhaps a vaccine could be developed from the virus that would protect people from getting RA.

MIND VS. BODY

RA may be caused by worry and stress. Doctors studying it found that several things could set off an attack of arthritis, or possibly the disease itself. These include infection, physical exposure, an injury directly to a joint, a weakened physical state, and emotional disturbances. One study created a "life chart" for patients with RA, who were asked to keep track of the onset of their attacks. The chart was reviewed to see if there was any relationship between the attacks and some stressful event. In 62 percent, a relationship was found.

HOW TO CREATE YOUR OWN LIFE CHART

Episodes of arthritis can be triggered by stress. Hans Selye, M.D., Ph.D., a noted authority on stress and disease, has described stress as the way your body responds to any demand. These demands or "stressing events" have specific effects, both physical and mental, which require some sort of change in your body.

Dr. Selye points out that stressful events need not be negative. In fact, any change in your emotional, environmental, or physical world can evoke a reaction. Events as exciting as a vacation, a child's wedding, or the purchase of a new car can create stress just as problems at work, an auto accident, or the breakup of an important relationship can. And if you suffer from arthritis, your reaction to the event can result in inflammation, with its accompanying redness, swelling, fever, malaise, heat, and pain.

We think the relationship between stressful events and arthritis episodes is important, so we've worked out a diary to help you keep track of them. Keep the diary for a year. Write down each day's events and any arthritic symptoms you experience. Some days you may have no entries, while on others you may have several. Each person and each day is different.

We have filled in the diary for one month's time to give an example of how to use it. Once you have completed the diary, look for patterns and consistencies. Did your fingers become sore three days after your salary review and also three days after your father took ill? Do positive events cause a different reaction than negative events? Does the degree of reaction change when you've had several stressful days back to back? Do the pains occur in the same areas over and over again?

It is impossible to eliminate all stress from your life, but you can adjust your reaction to it. Arnold Fox, M.D., an expert on stress and nutrition, feels that it is not the event but the way you react to the event that causes physical problems. Once you see how your life events affect your arthritis, try to concentrate on coping better.

In another study of 293 patients, 49 percent discovered that physical and/or emotional stress set off their attacks. The stress in men was job related, in women it was a combination of occupation and family worries. The study specifi-

Table 1:   **YOUR LIFE CHART**

Date	Stress Trigger	Arthritis Onset
8/1	Dental visit	
8/2	Forgot wedding anniversary Husband quits job	Severe morning stiffness
8/3	Sister engaged	
8/4	- - - - -	
8/5	Company picnic, little sleep	
8/6	Job interview for husband	Swollen right knee, very painful
8/7	- - - - -	
8/8	Dog delivers 11 puppies	
8/9	Father into hospital	Malaise
8/10	Friends visit from out of town with 3 children	
8/11	- - - - -	
8/12	Confirmed travel plans for 2 weeks vacation	Sore and swollen left hand
8/13	- - - - -	
8/14	Got bonus at work	
8/15	Bought new couch	
8/16	- - - - -	Sore wrist and elbow of left arm
8/17	- - - - -	
8/18	Dinner guests Missed period	
8/19	- - - - -	
8/20	- - - - -	Node develops on left elbow
8/21	- - - - -	

8/22	Make 5-hour drive Get little sleep	
8/23	– – – – –	
8/24	Make return 5-hour trip	
8/25	– – – – –	Fever, persistent ache in left knee and hand
8/26	– – – – –	
8/27	– – – – –	
8/28	– – – – –	

cally noted that when RA occurred in women over 40, it was often stress related.

Yet a third study showed that people with RA were a "decent lot" but tended to bottle up their feelings. Another revealed that people who are out-and-out psychotic *never* have RA. And in one study of eight identical twins—one of each pair with arthritis, one without—80 percent revealed that psychological stress had been part of their lives just before the onset of the disease. The twins without arthritis had no stress.

PARASITIC INFECTION

British physician Roger Wyburn-Mason says he knows the cause of RA. And the cure.

He says that RA is caused by a free-living protozoan (a parasitic amoeba) that can live indefinitely in the tissues of its host. Dr. Wyburn-Mason has found this parasite in the tissues of all patients with RA. Moreover, he says you can cure the disease by killing the protozoan with drugs.

His theory is that many people have a low-grade pathogenic amoeba infection in their intestines and bowels. Perhaps half of all people living in England, and as many as 70 to 80 percent of all people living in the southern United States, have these infections. He believes that a healthy liver with good bile function keeps the infection down, so that people seem to be in good health. However, should a person's resistance become low, the infection can spread to the joints and blood.

The medical community has not paid Dr. Wyburn-Mason much heed. Yet, he is a well-known doctor who has worked on both sides of the Atlantic. While serving as a lecturer and visiting professor at Yale University, he was one of the first investigators to describe the relationship between cancer and herpes.

In his work with arthritis, he isolated an amoeba from the body tissues of patients with rheumatoid disease. He found the organism could be killed by using the drug clotrimazole. However, the drug is very expensive ($500 per month for treatments) and very toxic. Its side effects include gastric bleeding, nausea, vomiting, diarrhea, cystitis, and skin rashes.

Dr. Wyburn-Mason is currently working with drugs that are less harsh, and awaiting test results.

If you think you may have RA (see It's Time to See Your Doctor, If—), consult your doctor as soon as possible. Once RA damages the joints, they cannot repair themselves. The trick is to get the disease diagnosed and under control very early, to minimize the damage to your joints.

When you go to the doctor he or she will take your

IT'S TIME TO SEE YOUR DOCTOR, IF—

you have:

- pain and stiffness on arising
- pain, tenderness, or swelling in one or more joints
- recurrence of pain, especially if it involves more than one joint
- recurrence of pain in the neck, lower back, knees, and other joints.

While rheumatic disease is often mild, it can recur and become chronic. If you have experienced any of these symptoms, it's time to see your doctor.

medical history and examine your joints for swelling, heat, loss of motion, and possibly early signs of deformity. Next, you'll be asked to have some laboratory tests done. Usually, these include a urinalysis, a complete blood count, a sed rate test, a test for the rheumatoid factor in your blood, perhaps an examination of joint fluid (usually taken from the knee), and X rays of key joints. See the Glossary for a complete explanation of these tests.

Juvenile Rheumatoid Arthritis

One day Mitchel Greene, age 11, developed a sore knee. It hurt a lot, and very quickly became very swollen. His parents took one look at it and rushed him to the Emergency Room at the local hospital. The doctor on duty there assumed the swelling was the result of an injury, and simply drained the water off the knee to restore it to its normal size and flexibility.

Mitchel didn't remember falling or doing anything else that might have hurt his knee. But then, kids are kids; they're always banging into something or playing too roughly.

After a day or two, the incident was forgotten. Mitchel was getting around well, going bowling, and playing with his friends. Business as usual. Then, almost one month to the day after his first bout with a sore knee, it happened again. Mitchel's knee got hot and swollen, and hurt like mad. This time his parents took him to the family doctor who, in turn, referred them to a rheumatologist in the nearest city. The rheumatologist ordered blood tests and examined Mitchel carefully. The final diagnosis: juvenile rheumatoid arthritis (JRA). For more than two years, Mitchel suffered with pains in his large joints, particularly his knees and shoulders. He took a heavy dose of aspirin daily for ten months. Sometimes he wore a device to immobilize his knee, and sometimes he used crutches. But he always went to school, and even kept up with his bowling league. During Mitchel's illness, the symptoms would mysteriously come and go. One day they went permanently.

Today Mitchel is 16. He no longer suffers from joint pain, and the bout with JRA seems to have left no permanent after-effects. It did not slow his growth or deform his joints.

Table 2:	JUVENILE RHEUMATOID ARTHRITIS (JRA)			
Type	Percent all JRA	Number Girls to Boys	Age of Onset	Outstanding Symptoms
Systemic JRA	20	8–10	any age	Joint pain; high fever; rash; swollen liver, spleen, lymph nodes; inflammation of the lung membrane; inflammation of the sac surrounding the heart; abdominal pain; high white blood cell count; iritis; severe anemia
Polyarticular JRA (Joint pain; affects 4 or more joints)				
Rheumatoid Factor+	30	6–1	8 or older	Nodules; low-grade fever; anemia
Rheumatoid Factor−	10	8–1	any age	Low-grade fever; mild anemia
Pauciarticular JRA (Joint pain; affects 4 or fewer joints, not usually symmetrically)				
Young Onset Type	25	7–1	5 or younger	Rheumatoid Factor tests do not apply; eye problems in 50% of cases
Older Onset Type	15	1–10	8 or older	Rheumatoid Factor test negative; affects hips often; genetic marker shows in 50% of cases; family history of iridocyclitis (an eye disorder) and ankylosing spondylitis

Mitchel Greene was pretty lucky. He had one of the milder forms of JRA. Doctors designate the disease as any form of arthritis that hits someone younger than 16. About 100,000 kids in the United States have been diagnosed as having JRA, a disease that comes in three forms. One type affects only a few joints, and, except for joint pain, causes no further feelings of sickness. Called *pauciarticular JRA,* it is the mildest of all forms. However, it can affect the eyes, causing a disease of the iris (the colored part).

The second type usually affects four or more joints, and is called *polyarticular JRA.* Kids with this type of JRA usually suffer with a low-grade fever, may develop nodules under the skin, and sometimes become anemic.

The third type is *systemic JRA,* which can hit any number of joints or just one. The child with systemic JRA can develop a high fever, a salmon-colored rash that looks like measles, inflammation of the iris in the eye, enlargement of the liver and spleen, and pain in the upper spine.

Sean Barrett is such a child. Now 11, he's suffered with the disease since he was 2. He has the distinction of being the youngest child in the country to have had a total hip replacement—at the age of 9.

"When I first realized he was sick, it was because he was terribly cranky and cried when he woke up in the morning after a nap," his mother Barbara explains. "Of course, I didn't realize it then, but he was suffering from morning stiffness.

"At the beginning of his illness, he ran a high fever of 103° almost daily for two months. We treated him with baby aspirin, but it took a while to work. He's been on aspirin for years, and at one time had bleeding ulcers. Fortunately, he's had no problem with his stomach for the last two years.

"Sean has a very severe form of JRA, in the 98th percentile of severity. He spends one or two months each year in the hospital. His growth has been severely stunted. And, even after the hip replacement, he spends most of his day sitting," she says.

Yet, Sean is a regular kid. He goes to public school, has lots of friends, and is even running for president of the student body. He's been labeled both handicapped and gifted. (He learned to read when he was three.) Sometimes he wishes that God would wave a magic wand and just make the disease go away, but generally he accepts his physical limitations.

He ignores Little League, and instead polishes his chess game—for which he's won trophies. He hopes to be a sportscaster when he grows up. "He can do it, too," Barbara says. "He talks all day long!"

Sean's doctor believes that the illness is the result of a genetic predisposition to the disease.

And that is the opinion much of the medical establishment has arrived at. Roger Hollister, M.D., a specialist in JRA at the National Jewish Hospital/National Asthma Center in Denver, Colorado, says, "Using recent tools, we have found that kids with JRA share a similar genetic background. But the cause of the disease is not entirely genetic. For example, you can have two identical twins with identical genetic backgrounds—and one will have JRA but the other won't. It seems there is a second factor that sparks the disease in the genetically predisposed. Perhaps it's a virus, or possibly something from the environment.

"I personally believe that a virus is the trigger, but there have been a lot of studies in this area, and no proof found. Sometimes parents ask if pollutants or food additives or chemicals could be the trigger. But I don't think so because these diseases have been around a lot longer than food additives or pollution. Research will give us the answer soon; we are very close right now."

The cause of JRA, then, is somehow linked to our heredity. Yet, unlike height and eye color, JRA need not be an unchangeable predetermined trait. Some kids simply outgrow JRA, while others will not. Dr. Hollister says, "Those with pauciarticular form of JRA have the best chance to outgrow the disease. Usually in the teen years. Kids with polyarticular form are given a blood test for the presence of a rheumatoid factor. Those with a negative factor have a better chance of outgrowing the disease than those with a positive factor. And the kids with the systemic JRA find the high fever and rash last about a year, then disappear. Some eventually grow out of the disease, but others switch, developing polyarticular arthritis, with joint pain as the main symptom."

While some doctors have advanced theories that stress,

like that caused by parental divorce, can kick off the disease, Dr. Hollister disagrees. He thinks that those under stress just may be more aware of their pain, or give in to it more readily. However, he does not believe that stress—whether from a broken home, a move to a new house, or final exams—causes JRA.

Systemic Lupus Erythematosus

Systemic lupus erythematosus is a disease of unknown origin, with no known cure, which attacks the body's connective tissue, or collagen. For reasons which are not understood, people with systemic lupus produce antibodies to their own tissue, which results in damage to one or more of their internal organs.

The disease can affect the skin, kidneys, nervous system, and internal membranes. Its unique feature is a rash, shaped like a butterfly, that spreads across the nose and cheeks. Joint pain also occurs in more than 90 percent of those who have lupus, but arthritis deformities are rare.

In most cases, lupus is characterized by alternate remissions and relapses, which can be brief, but may continue for extended lengths of time.

For every man who gets lupus, eight or nine women do, most of them between the ages of 20 and 40. It is not a rare disease, but affects 1 in every 1,000 people.

As recently as 17 years ago, the disease was usually fatal. Today, with the use of long-term cortisone therapy, the disease can often be held in check. Unfortunately, long-term treatment with cortisone causes numerous side effects, some of which are themselves fatal.

Susan Laird, a young woman from Connecticut, suffered with severe lupus, but managed to overcome it in just a bit more than a year.

"The first inkling I had of my illness was in the spring of 1977. My symptom was dizziness that came upon me without warning, with such severity and violence I thought I must be having a heart attack.

"The worst of it lasted about 20 minutes and then, although it abated, it never went away. For the next four months I was dizzy, and often nauseated as well, from the moment I got up in the morning until I went to bed at night.

"Meanwhile, the doctors did brain scans, EEG's, EKG's, blood workups, neurological tests, a five-hour glucose tolerance test, and assorted ear examinations. When they ran out of tests, they started repeating ones already done.

"They gave me drugs for my nerves, drugs to stop the dizziness, drugs for nausea, antihypertensive drugs, diuretics, and finally a drug for myasthenia gravis (one of the many misdiagnoses the doctors made along the way).

"All the while, I continued to deteriorate.

"Physically, I was getting weaker and weaker. Some days my energy quota was spent by the time I walked downstairs in the morning and let the dog out. Other days I would drive to work, only to eke out just enough energy to turn around and return home to spend the rest of the day flat on my back in bed."

Eight months and five doctors after her first attack, Susan was diagnosed as having systemic lupus. She was given a prescription for cortisone, which she ignored. Instead, under alternative medical supervision, she fasted, rested, discovered several hidden food allergies, and eliminated those foods from her diet, which she then supplemented with vitamins and minerals. Fifteen months after the diagnosis of lupus, Susan's blood tests were normal and she felt like her healthy old self again.

Susan warns, however, that the knowledge of having a chronic disease with no known cure can be as emotionally painful as the arthritic joints are physically painful.

"There is depression associated with having been struck by a supposedly incurable disease, and despair at feeling trapped between dead and alive, not really one or the other. A psychologist I was seeing, a bit of a health nut himself, hypnotized me to help me deal with the anxiety, taught me self-hypnosis to relax, and listened hour after hour as I described ad nauseam the disease's debilitating effects," she says.

Lupus is usually diagnosed by a blood test, which reveals abnormal autoantibodies, signs that the body is attacking itself. The primary symptom of lupus is pain. The joints hurt because the synovial membrane is inflamed, and the pain is fairly steady. However, the disease tends to lessen in severity over a period of years.

Psoriatic Arthritis

Arthritis is a common disease. Psoriasis is a common disease. Therefore, it shouldn't come as any big surprise that some people with arthritis also may have psoriasis. However, in addition to the chance coexistence of the two diseases in the same individual, there's also a totally distinct form of arthritis—psoriatic arthritis—that is common among those who suffer with psoriasis.

The association between psoriasis and arthritis was noted in medical literature more than 150 years ago. However, psoriatic arthritis wasn't recognized as a separate disease until 1927. It differs from RA in that usually only the small joints of the fingers and toes are affected. Often the nails and nail beds are pitted with psoriasis, and the fingers can swell to look like sausages. In addition, the fever, fatigue, and morning stiffness are less severe than in RA, there are no nodules under the skin, and remission is more frequent.

Usually, a person with this odd form of arthritis develops psoriasis first. In fact, it may take 10 to 12 years before the joints begin to ache. And, according to a Mayo Clinic study, those with the most severe skin problems are the likely candidates for arthritis. Once the disease is established, both the skin and joint problems come and go simultaneously.

Because psoriatic arthritis runs in families, doctors have assumed that heredity can make you susceptible. This assumption is supported by a study of tissues taken from people with psoriatic arthritis. Lab tests turned up suspicious antibodies that don't appear in people who have just plain psoriasis.

The arthritis is inflammatory. Treating it involves treating the psoriasis, getting enough rest, and gently exercising the inflamed joints. At the Washington Hospital Center in Washington, D.C., patients were treated with PUVA, a combination of ultraviolet light waves and chemicals. Some patients with psoriatic arthritis involving their small joints got much relief from the treatments. Their skin cleared and their joints stopped aching. However, those who had problems in their spine, rather than their joints, didn't do as well. In fact, the problems seemed to be independent, with back pain and rash operating on different wavelengths, so to speak. The doctors at Washington Hospital Center therefore have speculated that psoriatic arthritis may actually be broken into two broad groups—of the spine and of the joints.

* * *

These many, varied types of RA present a complex jigsaw puzzle for medical science. The one definite unifying link is inflammation of the synovial membrane. However, most doctors also feel that a second link is the hereditary "weakness" that may allow some other factors—like a virus—to spark the disease. Causes and cures are theories. The key to living with RA is to outsmart it and outlive it. Early diagnosis and early treatment can limit permanent damage to the joints. Exercise and a hopeful, determined outlook can help you to live fully, while you control the disease.

4

ABOUT GOUT
... AND PSEUDOGOUT

Oh! When I have the gout I feel as if I was walking on my eyeballs.

**Sydney Smith, English writer and Anglican priest
(1771–1845)**

When asked what he knew about gout, the editor of a well-known health newsletter asked, "Is that still with us?"

Sure enough, it is. But the editor isn't alone in assuming that gout went out with powdered wigs and satin knickers. It's a disease long associated with royalty and its excesses—gluttony and debauchery among them. It's probably best exemplified by Henry VIII, who ate, drank and (some think) wed too often.

Sorry to say, gout lasted beyond most kings and kingdoms, surviving to torture ordinary mortals who never gave even one thought to the Divine Right of Kings. In fact, in the United States today, about 1,600,000 people suffer with this exquisitely painful malady.

Most people don't think of gout as a form of arthritis, but it really is. The term was introduced 700 years ago, and is derived from the Latin word *gutta*, which means *a drop*. It reflects the early belief that a poison fell drop by drop into a joint, causing swelling, redness, and pain. If we substitute the word *crystal* for the word *gutta,* the old definition would be correct. The disease, you see, is caused by crystals that accumulate in the joints, creating great pain and swelling. Often the crystals—which are made of sodium urate—also collect in the cartilage, in the kidneys, and in growths called tophi that develop under the skin.

Gout is primarily a man's disease, although women become somewhat more susceptible after menopause. Generally, it doesn't strike men under 30. But for those who are susceptible, the fifth decade of life is the most common time to come down with the disease.

Gout is caused by an inborn error in metabolism. Tell *that* to your friends who have been accusing you of dining nightly on a joint of ox washed down with a flagon of claret. Sure, diet and alcohol come into play where gout is concerned. But take two men of identical age, give them both a rich, boozy diet, and only the guy with the inborn problem will get gout. (The other fellow may die of a heart attack, but he won't get gout!)

Here's how it works. If you have gout, your body either produces too much uric acid, or it produces just the right amount but doesn't excrete enough of it. Some people have both problems—too much uric acid and too little excretion. Therefore, above certain levels it begins to form into microscopic crystals of sodium urate. Shaped like needles and just as sharp, they prick themselves into joint tissue. For some reason, the joint of the big toe is particularly susceptible.

Gout actually can begin years before your first attack, with a growing level of uric acid in the blood. This condition is called *hyperuricemia,* and is a precondition of gout. Interestingly, hyperuricemia is related to both great intelligence and great anxiety. Indeed, if you review the famous people in history who have suffered with gout, you'll see they were no dummies. They include: Achilles, Oedipus, Ulysses, Erasmus the Scholar, Michelangelo, Leonardo da Vinci, Samuel Johnson, John Milton, Alexander the Great, Isaac Newton, Martin Luther, John Calvin, James I, the aforementioned Henry VIII, Horace Walpole, Charles Darwin, and Ben Franklin, among others.

As the levels of uric acid build in the blood, the person with hyperuricemia feels perfectly well. Then, one fine day,

Table 3:   **GUIDELINES FOR A LOW-PURINE DIET**

Foods Likely to Induce Gout (Avoid at all times)

Approximate purine content ranges from 150 to 1,000 milligrams each per 3½-ounce serving.

Anchovies	Liver
Asparagus	Meat extracts
Brains	Mincemeat
Consomme	Mushrooms
Gravies	Mussels
Heart	Sardines
Herring	Sweetbread
Kidney	

Foods That May Contribute to Gout (Limit to just 1 serving daily)

Approximate purine content ranges from 50 to 150 milligrams each per 3½-ounce serving.

Beans, dry	Peas, dry
Cauliflower	Poultry*
Fish*	Seafood
Lentils	Spinach
Meats*	Whole-grain cereals
Oatmeal	Yeast

SOURCES: Adapted from *Normal and Therapeutic Nutrition*, by Corinne H. Robinson and Marilyn R. Lawler (New York: Macmillan Co., 1977).

Human Nutrition, by Benjamin T. Burton (New York: McGraw-Hill, 1976).

*Limit these foods to 3-ounce servings, 5 days a week.

or even more likely, night, gout attacks one or more joints. The attack may be brought on by any number of things. Breaking in a new pair of shoes can do it. Or going for a long walk. It also can be triggered by a rich diet, alcohol, surgery, or certain drugs like liver extracts, insulin, or even penicillin.

The attack can last from 3 to 11 days, during which time the joint is swollen and dusky red. Inside the joint, the urate crystals have started chemical reactions in the joint fluid that result in inflammation. The cells of the body's defense system rush to the sore joint, creating even more congestion. In addition, the powerful enzymes they release can make the inflammation more painful and longer lasting. After the attack, the joint simply returns to normal.

Fortunately, about half of all people who have the first attack of gout never have a second. However, others can expect intermittent attacks which (fortunately) yield quickly to medical treatment.

Modern medicine has shown that the reason for the excess uric acid that creates all this pain is found in the body's inability to metabolize purines. During cell breakdown and replacement, purines are metabolized into uric acid. Indeed, eating purine-rich foods has long been associated with cases of gout. These foods include organ meats, anchovies, sardines, and herring. See Table 3.

So, while the basis of disease is inherited, it can be controlled to a great extent by diet and lifestyle. Doctors noted that during and immediately after both World Wars I and II, gout was uncommon in Europe. However, when a variety of protein-rich foods again became widely available, more people got gout. The same thing is happening today in Japan. As the Japanese have adopted a more Western diet, their protein consumption has doubled. And the incidence of gout has increased accordingly.

Another discovery of modern medicine is the link between gout and alcohol. Back in the eighteenth century, most people knew that rich meals and gout were somehow related. Many people suspected alcohol, too, but it wasn't until the 1960s that anyone pinned down the connection.

At the Clinical Research Center of the Presbyterian University Hospital in Pittsburgh, Pennsylvania, patients were given both purine-rich meals and alcohol to see how it would affect their gout. Working with six men and one woman, Gerald Rodnan, M.D., placed the patients on a purine-free diet to stabilize the urate levels in their blood. Then, the patients were given a large evening meal, containing two to five grams of purine. First, the meals were eaten without wine or spirits, and the patient's uric acid levels rose somewhat. But when alcohol was given along with the meal, the urate levels rose sharply. In some cases, they almost doubled their previous level. Six of the seven patients had acute attacks of gout within the next four days.

And so we have an airborn condition that makes a person vulnerable to certain foods and alcohol. In addition, several diseases are associated with gout, including Down's syndrome, lead poisoning, some bone marrow disorders, a form of diabetes called *nephrogenic diabetes insipidus,* psoriasis, and chronic kidney disorders.

Gout can be quite diverse, attacking one or several joints. The big toe is so often the target that this form of gout has earned its own name: *podagra.* However, the disease also can attack tendon sheaths and bursae, as well as joints. In addition to joint problems, some people with gout also form kidney stones. Others develop tophi, growths that appear over the body's bony knobs or along the outer edges of the ears. The tophi are made of sodium urate crystals.

Horace Walpole, an English author and politician of the eighteenth century, suffered with gout all his life. In a letter to his friend Horace Mann, he described his gouty tophi this way:

> A finger of each hand has been pouring out a hail of chalk-stones and liquid chalk; and the first finger, which I hoped exhausted, last week opened again and threw out a cascade of the latter, exactly with the effort of a pipe that bursts in the streets.

Gout generally has four stages. The first is symptom-free, the second is a gout attack, the third is the period between attacks, and the fourth is chronic tophaceous gout— where the attacks no longer come and go. Instead, they come and stay. Walpole most likely spent the better part of his pain-filled life in this fourth stage.

Fortunately, the gout of today is just a pale shadow of the "disease of kings." It has been tamed by a medicine that can dissolve the crystals that cause inflammation. And, as we have seen, the crystal formation itself can be prevented or moderated by carefully following the proper diet.

If your doctor suspects you have gout, he will draw off some joint fluid, and examine it for the telltale needle-shaped urate crystals. You also may require a blood test to measure the level of uric acid in your system.

If you're diagnosed as having gout, you may be asked to lose weight and lay off foods high in purine content. If you have developed tophi, they can be removed surgically or dissolved with medication.

In any case, the outlook for a person with gout is excellent. Despite the disease's royal-pain past, its present and future are undistinguished.

Pseudogout—A First Cousin

Pseudogout is a condition that closely resembles gout, even to the crystals that lodge in the joints. Its causes, however, are different from gout—and the crystals are made of a different substance entirely.

What happens when you have this disease, which is also called *chondrocalcinosis,* is that crystals made of calcium salts develop and gravitate to the joints. Unlike gout, however, the disease generally strikes older people rather than those in their middle years. Also unlike gout's abrupt attacks, pseudogout sometimes comes on gradually. And where gout has an affinity for the small joints such as those in your toe or wrist, pseudogout usually affects the larger joints, especially the knee. Finally, where gout strikes 20 men for every woman, the odds are almost even for either sex to develop pseudogout.

An attack of pseudogout can be brought on by an injury or surgery or both. Alcohol, a rich diet, or too strenuous exercise seem to have little to do with the onset. The condition is also found as a secondary result of a more serious disease, particularly hyperparathyroidism, Wilson's disease, and diabetes.

No one knows what sort of metabolic malfunction is responsible for pseudogout. What medical science does know is that these calcium crystals aggravate the synovial lining of the joint, causing inflammation. The joint becomes stiff, warm, and swollen. And it hurts. Sometimes the skin over the joint becomes red. Once an attack kicks off, it will not reach its peak intensity for 12 to 36 hours. The most common complaint of people with pseudogout is that of tossing in bed, trying to find comfort, or at least a bit of relief.

There is no known way to stop the crystals from depositing in the joints. However, one simple, effective treatment is to draw off some fluid from the sore joint, taking the crystals along with it.

Gout and pseudogout, which have plagued humanity throughout the ages, were never thought to be part of arthritis. In fact, one famous saying—this from Philip Dormer Stanhope, the Earl of Chesterfield back in the eighteenth century—distinguishes the two diseases not only as distinctly different from arthritis (which he calls "rheumatism"), but also related to social class. He said, "Gout . . . is the distemper of the gentleman; whereas the rheumatism is the distemper of the hackney-coachman or chairman, who is obliged to be out in all weathers and at all hours."

Sorry, Lord Chesterfield, but the years have proven you wrong on both counts. It's the diet, not the pocketbook, that makes the difference. And it's the internal climate rather than the atmospheric that takes the toll. Either way, today's gout sufferer—gentleman, coachman, housewife, or movie star— can take comfort in the fact that control of the disease rests mainly in using common sense.

DR. JOHNSON'S DISEASE . . . BY ANY NAME, IT'S GOUT
by Calvin Trillin

I suppose you've heard by now that I had the gout. Everybody seems to know. No, I don't want to hear about your grandfather's gout. With the possible exception of your grandmother, nobody is less interested in hearing about your grandfather than I am. No, gout does not make people ill tempered. I have nothing against your grandfather—although I must admit that even before the onset of my own affliction, stories concerning the inflammation of his joints would not have been high on my list of compelling narratives. The reason I'm adamant right now about not wanting to discuss your grandfather is that the association of gout with grandfathers— particularly grandfathers who look like Charles Laughton—is symptomatic of a view of gout that we gout sufferers consider a very large pain in the foot.

Don't deny it. Charles Laughton is precisely the sort of person you had in mind. I know that from the smile my wife had on her face when she guessed that I might have the gout—after having dismissed, without anything approaching a scientific inquiry, my theory that I might be suffering from the effects of a tarantula bite. I heard that Charles Laughton echo in the voice of my doctor, who took one look at my foot and said, "Looks like a touch of the gout, old boy." I know the picture he had in his mind. Some bloated old Tory sunk into a leather armchair in a musty gentlemen's club, resting one foot on a gout-stool as he tries to maneuver the other foot into position to kick at a passing waiter. Don't tell me: You were just about to say that gout is the disease of the rich and distinguished. I know what you really mean. You really mean that people who have the gout are rich enough to guzzle vintage port and distinguished by a tendency to let cigar ashes dribble onto their vests as they doze off in the middle of the afternoon. Don't deny it.

Your attitude is the reason I decided that there had to be a serious effort to reeducate the public on the subject of gout—which, of course, is not the name our affliction will go by once the reeducation effort is in high gear.

"We need to come up with a new name," I told my wife. "Maybe something that sounds breezy, like the names they use these days for new brands of cigarettes."

"How about Glutton's Syndrome?" my wife said.

I explained to her that according to modern medical theory, gout is more likely to have to do with heredity than with diet, although just to be safe I have always steered clear of mung beans and broccoli. Then it occurred to me that we might name the disease after one or another of its most renowned sufferers, such as Dr. Samuel Johnson—the eighteenth-century literary figure, not the oral surgeon.

"What about calling it Johnson's Disease?" I asked.

"That's a dumb name," she said. "People will think it's named after Lyndon Johnson. They'll think the symptoms include a mad compulsion to bomb Orientals."

Dumb! I wasn't going to bring this up, but, as it happens, studies suggest a correlation between Dr. Johnson's Disease (formerly gout) and high intelligence. Name three dummies who have ever had Dr. Johnson's Disease. See! The reeducation campaign is in high gear already.

In planning the campaign, I got off on the wrong foot—a phrase, I must say, that still makes me wince, even though some little pills the doctor gave me cleared up my symptoms (or coincided with the gradual neutralizing of the tarantula venom I had absorbed). The false association of gout with the Blimps had made me obsessed with distinguishing the sort of people who actually do get Dr.

Johnson's Disease (Galileo, for instance, and Richard the Lionhearted) from the sort of people who don't. Roy Cohn, the New York Bar's best-known limousine-chaser, had just thrown the annual birthday celebration that I have always thought of as the Foxhole Party, since it brings together all of the most prominent people you wouldn't want to have in the next foxhole, and I became preoccupied with proving that the sort of people who contract Dr. Johnson's Disease would not be in attendance. As a public service, the *Soho News,* of blessed memory, usually had a reporter on hand at the Foxhole Party to note the names of guests as they arrived—the way the F.B.I. stations someone at the cemetery to check out the mourners at a mob funeral—and I was poring over the list when my wife told me I was wasting my time trying to prove that no sufferer of Dr. Johnson's Disease would attend a party held at a disco.

"That little jig that Hitler danced when he heard about the fall of France would have been impossible for a man with Dr. Johnson's Disease," I informed her.

"I think you need professional help," she said.

I tried to get some from a friend in the public relations business. He suggested that we build a campaign around television commercials featuring Bruce Jenner, the decathlon champion, and have as our first big fund-raiser a benefit performance of that new film *I'm Dancing as Fast as I Can.* The commercials would show Jenner just barely outrunning and outjumping some beach-boy type, and would then cut to the locker room, where Jenner says to the beach boy, "Hey, you're not bad for a guy with the gout."

"We call it Dr. Johnson's Disease, or D.J.D., these days, Bruce," the beach boy says, with diction that makes it obvious he is not a beach boy but maybe an associate professor of classics. "And with proper medication, people who suffer from it can lead full and productive lives."

You can be assured that I rejected that campaign out of hand. I don't want people to think that those of us who have D.J.D. do not suffer. We want respect, sure, but not at the cost of losing sympathy. D.J.D. hurts. Sometimes, I had to keep my foot up on a stool. Sometimes, I got, well, out of sorts, which you would get too if your foot hurt and you weren't allowed any wine as long as you were taking little pills. Sometimes, what bothered me most about my foot hurting was that I couldn't use it to drop-kick a cat. Sometimes the medication made me doze off. You suspected as much, didn't you? Don't deny it.

SOURCE: "Uncivil Liberties," by Calvin Trillin, *The Nation*, March 27, 1982. Copyright © 1982. Used with permission of Nation Associates, Inc.

5

ARTHRITIS THAT ISN'T

Suppose, as you twist the car key in the ignition, you discover that your right wrist is very sore and stiff. Suppose it hurts, too, when you lift a gallon jug of cider. Or when you push a revolving door, hang clothes on the washline, try to do push-ups, or turn a tight screw. Should you automatically assume you have arthritis?

Not at all. Some people develop these identical symptoms from fairly minor causes, like playing the game Space Invaders for too many hours, or overexerting on the tennis or racquetball court.

In other words, arthritis isn't always the culprit that causes aches and creaks in the joints. In fact, there is a whole group of diseases that mimic arthritis. And while these conditions may cause just as much pain, they technically are not arthritis because the source of the pain is not inside the joint itself. Instead, the cause is often inflammation found in adjacent areas, such as in the ligaments and tendons that string the muscles and bones to the joints. Sometimes the problem develops in the vertebrae of the spine—also technically not a joint. These conditions often result from trauma, overwork, or abuse. Others actually are complications of a more serious disease, and go away when the primary disease clears up.

This group of arthritislike diseases includes ankylosing spondylitis, arthritis associated with inflammatory bowel disease, Reiter's disease, traumatic arthritis, tenosynovitis, and the basic bad back. The individual diseases can range from minor annoyances to major debilitating conditions. Because they are so different, let's consider each one separately.

Ankylosing Spondylitis

Humans have been plagued by this disease since at least the third century B.C. If it's any consolation, it also strikes horses and monkeys and has even been found in the remains of prehistoric crocodiles. Old-timers may know it as Marie-Strumpell disease, named after the nineteenth-century scientists who first described it fully.

Ankylosing spondylitis is a fairly common back problem among young men. While it does affect women, it is not usual and generally remains very mild. The disease most often begins when a person is quite young—possibly as young as 15. However, it usually is not diagnosed until about the age of 40.

The condition is popularly called "poker spine," a very appropriate nickname. In very bad cases of ankylosing spondylitis, bone forms between the vertebrae of the spine, eventually fusing the spine, skull, ribs, and hips into one long bone that cannot bend. Hence the name.

If you have ankylosing spondylitis, chances are very remote that you will ever develop true poker spine. Most cases are not so severe. Generally, what happens is that you begin to feel pain in the lower back, along with some stiffness. The beginning of the disease is not dramatic. In fact, you may hardly notice it. As time goes on, the pain grows stronger so that you ache and feel stiff for several days in a row. Then, quite magically, you feel better. This pattern of sickness/wellness repeats.

Usually, the disease moves up the spine. In about one-third of the cases, some joints in the arms and legs occasionally become inflamed, too. While you're aching, you also tend to lose your appetite (and some weight) and may run a low-grade fever. Generally speaking, you feel your absolute worst when you get out of bed in the morning.

As the disease spreads, it often affects the sacroiliac—that is, the joint in the lower back where that little triangular bone just above the buttocks meets the hip bones. It also may develop in the fibrous joints where the ribs meet the backbone, both front and back. As these joints become inflamed, fibrous tissue grows out of the synovial membrane and into the cartilage that lines the joint. Eventually the joint space

57

becomes totally filled with this fibrous material. At the very same time, the bones *near* the joint also become inflamed and hardened. Ultimately, the joint space simply disappears. It turns into solid bone. In the spine itself, the vertebrae and disks also become united by bony growth.

Initially, this disease is painful. However, once the fusion has taken place, there is no more pain. Only stiffness remains. If the ribs and spine have become fused, deep breathing will be difficult because chest expansion has been limited. In very severe cases, the eyes can become inflamed, the aortic valve in the heart may not function properly, and cavities can develop in the lungs. These symptoms, however, are limited to very severe cases.

While the description of the disease sounds catastrophic, most people who have ankylosing spondylitis live normal, active lives. They usually have no trouble getting around and don't miss any more days from work than anybody else.

IT'S TIME TO SEE YOUR DOCTOR, IF—

- you have low-back pain that has lasted for more than three months and hasn't improved with rest
- your chest is painful, stiff, and doesn't expand fully
- you can't bend your lower back
- your eyes are inflamed, particularly in the area of the iris
- your family has a history of this disease.

The cause of ankylosing spondylitis apparently is heredity. More than half the people with the disease have others in their family with the same problem. The culprit is a gene labeled B27. Almost every white person with ankylosing spondylitis has been found to have this gene. It is less commonly found in people of other races.

Arthritis Associated with Inflammatory Bowel Disease

You'd think folks with intestinal problems have enough difficulty without the added burden of arthritis. Even so, in some forms of bowel disease, arthritis develops as a complication. The relationship between the two is murky. Medical science doesn't even know what causes the bowel problems, let alone why they are related to arthritis.

The two bowel diseases that piggyback arthritis are ulcerative colitis and regional enteritis, an umbrella term that includes Crohn's disease, granulomatous colitis, and transmural colitis. Those suffering with these problems tend to develop either ankylosing spondylitis or peripheral arthritis—that is, either arthritis affecting the spine or the joints in the limbs.

About 15 percent of all ulcerative colitis patients develop peripheral arthritis. It comes on suddenly, usually between the ages of 25 and 45. It tends to affect the knees and ankles most often, but can shift to other joints as well. An attack can last one or two months. However, despite the length of the attacks, they are not grave because they don't happen very often. For example, most patients with ulcerative colitis experience only two attacks of peripheral arthritis over a five-year span.

Spondylitis, too, often comes with colitis. In fact, the portion of the population that has ulcerative colitis has 100 times more cases of ankylosing spondylitis than the rest of the general public. And while this form of arthritis generally strikes 9 young men for every woman, bowel disease equalizes the sex distribution to 2.5 men to every woman.

The relationship between the two conditions has yet to be explained. However, one theory recently has been developed. It's been found that people who had an intestinal bypass operation to lose weight often developed arthritis. Apparently, the shortened bowel somehow allows arthritis to develop. Researchers working at the Germantown Medical Center in Philadelphia, Pennsylvania, have theorized that bacteria from the damaged bowel may be absorbed into the body, somehow kicking off an immune response that mistakenly destroys joint and connective tissue. Should this form of arthritis be caused by bacteria, scientists are sure an antibiotic can be developed to treat it.

Reiter's Disease

Named after the German doctor who described it way back in 1916, Reiter's disease is a pretty rare form of arthritis. Nevertheless, it is the second most common form among young men. (Ankylosing spondylitis is the first.) It is sometimes called the "soldier's disease" because it is most common among military personnel, particularly those stationed away from home. It seems to be transmitted by sexual intercourse, especially the extramarital kind. Doctors are at a loss to explain the relationship exactly, but note that Reiter's disease also follows an epidemic of dysentery. They therefore assume the disease to be the result of an infectious bacteria.

It is more than a disease of the joints. It also can involve the genitals and the eyes. The first symptom is not a stiff or sore joint, but rather superficial ulcers on the genitals and/or bloody diarrhea, later followed by joint aches and inflamed eyes. The joints most often affected are the hips and knees, but the fingers and toes sometimes get involved, too. Joints are usually not affected on both sides at the same time.

The exact cause of Reiter's disease is unknown, but most people who get the disease have an inherited predisposition that makes them susceptible to it. Almost everyone who catches Reiter's disease simply recovers completely, with little or no chance of a recurrence.

Traumatic Arthritis

Traumatic arthritis is the term used to describe a joint problem that has developed after trauma (like a sharp blow) or after a long period of abuse. It includes such diverse conditions as Space Invaders' wrist, along with housemaid's knee, tailor's bottom, slot machine tendinitis, and miner's elbow.

It is also defined as a problem in a spot near but not in the joint. Thus, the term traumatic arthritis also includes tendinitis, bursitis, and even strains and sore muscles. For the record, tendinitis is an inflammation of the tough cord that leads from the muscle to the joint; bursitis is an inflammation of a small sac found near the joint which provides lubrication; a strain is a torn or stretched ligament that leads to a joint; and a sore muscle is a sore muscle.

Fortunately, most cases of traumatic arthritis just clear up after a period of rest and refraining from whatever activity caused the problem in the first place. Unfortunately, when the "trauma" is an activity that is part of your job or daily life—even an activity as nonstrenuous as typing—the arthritis can become serious. For instance, osteoarthritis can develop in joints that are repeatedly traumatized. Often boxers will develop it in their wrists, or soccer players in their ankles. Sometimes, too, calcium deposits can form on the tendons, causing pain that can range from minor to stabbingly acute. This particular brand of arthritis can trouble even clerical workers or others who don't do strenuous physical labor.

Probably the most talked-about form of traumatic arthritis is tennis elbow. Found most frequently in middle-aged men, the problem is caused by an overextension of the wrist, repeated many times. The treatment is to switch games. (But not to Space Invaders!)

Tenosynovitis, the Tender Tendon

There is a condition where joint pain arises not from the joint or even from the tendons and ligaments, but rather from an inflammation of the tube through which the tendon passes. The medical name for this condition is *tenosynovitis*. While this inflammation can be caused by certain forms of arthritis such as rheumatoid arthritis or gout, it usually comes from trauma. The cause can be something as simple as new shoes that put unaccustomed pressure on the area of the Achilles tendon, or a brief but intense period of unusual activity. The symptoms are soreness and slight swelling, most often affecting the wrist or thumb. This form of tenosynovitis goes away by itself after a few days of rest.

There is, however, one type of tenosynovitis that is a bit

more mysterious and troublesome than most. It is called *carpal tunnel syndrome*.

With carpal tunnel syndrome, the people affected—usually middle-aged women—feel pain when they move their wrist. The pain often shoots down the fingers and up the forearm. In addition, the three middle fingers of the hand often feel numb and tingly, like when your hand "falls asleep."

The disease centers in the area where the bones and ligaments in your wrist form a tunnel through which pass the tendons and the nerves that make it possible for you to move your fingers and experience the sense of touch. According to Karl Folkers, Ph.D., director of the Institute for Biomedical Research at the University of Texas at Austin, an excess of fluid inside the carpal tunnel presses on the nerve, causing a tingling sensation in the fingertips.

Because the nerves are compressed, other more serious symptoms also may develop—painful elbows or shoulders and a very weak handgrip, to name a few. Sometimes symptoms are so severe people have to quit their jobs.

Those suffering with carpal tunnel syndrome sometimes mistake it for arthritis. It is not. In the past, the usual treatment for this condition was to rest the joint by putting a splint on it, or—all else failing—to relieve the pressure with surgery. Dr. Folkers, however, believes the cause of this syndrome is a vitamin B_6 deficiency. His experiments have shown that patients experience relief after taking vitamin B_6 supplements in the proper amounts. (See chapter 9 for specific details.)

The Basic Bad Back

Assorted back ailments afflict an estimated 70 million people in the United States each year. The causes can include muscle strain, poor posture, disk problems, and lax muscles, as well as arthritis. Here we will limit the discussion to types of back pain that are not caused by arthritis.

Everyday aches and pains in the back divide themselves into two main kinds—postural pain and dysfunctional pain. According to Lionel A. Walpin, M.D., clinical director of physical medicine and rehabilitation at Cedars-Sinai Medical Center in Los Angeles, California, "Postural pain comes on gradually. You may notice it developing after hunching over a desk for an hour or so. It's relieved, however, when you stand up and stretch or just change position. A person with pure postural pain is the one who has full mobility but who wakes up in the morning stiff and sore.

"With dysfunctional pain, on the other hand, you stand up, bend over and—*wham*—instant pain. With dysfunction (abnormal function of muscles and joints), you don't have full mobility. Also, only treating the pain in this case is not synonymous with recovery. You need to restore the normal strength, length, and flexibility of the dysfunctioning muscles and joints, too."

What is all this talk about muscles when it's the back that hurts? To understand the connection, you have to picture your spine. The spinal column is comprised of separate vertebrae that are stacked one atop the other, forming numerous joints where they meet. Muscles and ligaments keep those joints properly in place. The most important muscles for keeping the lower spine lined up are found in the abdomen. It's imperative these muscles are kept strong and healthy because they must help the spine bear quite a load. For instance, just sitting upright puts 300 pounds of pressure per square inch on the disks between your lumbar vertebrae (if you are of average weight); standing, 200 pounds; and even when lying flat on your back 100 pounds is still pressing on that area. If your abdominal muscles weaken, the normal curve of your lower back increases, and you get back pain.

In addition to improper alignment of the vertebrae, some back pains result from misplaced disks—little shock absorbers that separate the vertebrae. These disks contain a soft inner core and a tougher, more fibrous, outer portion. Under extreme pressure, the inner core can tear and push into the outer part, causing it to bulge and protrude outward from between the vertebrae. This "slipped" disk can press on nerves in the region and cause severe pain at the point of injury. The lumbar region, because of its curve, is particularly vulnerable to herniated disks, resulting, typically, in pain in the legs. (Injury to a cervical disk can result in pain in the arms.) While rest often will promote healing, many severely herniated disks require surgical removal.

Of course, misalignment of disks and vertebrae also can result from accidents and injuries. However, chronic problems can result if poor posture or repeated strain complicate the situation.

One final, seemingly unavoidable contributor to back pain is age. Some problems caused by age are strictly physical, while others result from the mental and emotional slump many of us experience as we grow older.

On the physical side, the problem is diminishing—that is, diminishing resilience, diminishing bone, and diminishing circulation. From age 20 on, the blood supply to the disks gradually stops. The disks become increasingly less resilient. At the point of greatest pressure—in the low back—the disk can wither away completely, leaving the vertebrae without their shock absorbers. A similar condition involves *osteoporosis,* a condition where the bones become less dense and strong. This condition often results from hormonal changes in women after menopause, from a calcium deficiency, or from prolonged use of cortisone. With osteoporosis, the spine actually shrinks.

Perhaps the most insidious cause of back pain, though, is the "Ole Rockin' Chair's Got Me" syndrome. Those suffering with the syndrome often complain of television reruns, tight waistbands, cold houses, and—you guessed it—an aching back. Once you decide that you're too old to get about, too stiff to be involved, too sore to care—the rocking chair doesn't just have you. It's trapped you! By spending day and night sitting, you lay waste to those important abdominal muscles that help keep your spine straight. Moreover, sitting too much decreases your circulation—making you a candidate for blood clots and varicose veins.

What's really odd is that sitting—usually thought of as a form of resting—can actually create fatigue. According to Arthur Weltman, Ph.D., a professor of exercise physiology at the University of Colorado, "A sedentary lifestyle has been widely cited as the most important cause of creeping obesity. Studies indicate that a lack of physical activity is more often the cause of overweight than is overeating. Active people— people who walk, cycle, jog, swim, or engage in a similar exercise for at least 30 minutes a day—have lower risk profiles for most diseases than sedentary people. And they also enjoy immediate benefits: firmer muscles, alertness, and energy instead of listlessness and fatigue; better and more restful sleep; and fun, recreation, and release."

Fun, it seems, is more important than you may at first think. People who are sedentary and inactive have few normal outlets to release their tensions. And tension itself has been known to cause back pains. It stays in the muscles, contracting them and making them stiff.

Find something you love to do, and do it. You may groan because it hurts a bit, but you'll be happier and healthier once you get on your feet and moving again.

Part 2
TAKING CHARGE

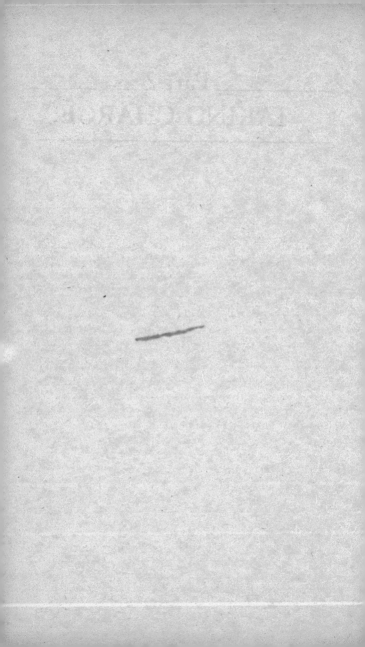

Introduction

So you have arthritis. If you're like most people with the disease, you probably feel you've been sentenced to a life term imprisoned in a body that hurts, a body that not only lost its fluid grace but barely moves, a body that has become an unwilling servant, a stranger, a traitor.

You probably feel angry and frustrated. And why not? These emotions are common among people with chronic diseases. They are, in fact, the feelings of a victim. If you view yourself as someone held hostage and tormented by pain, you are indeed a victim—even if your captor is not a person but a common disease. Like other captives or prisoners, people with arthritis sometimes feel powerless. The disease dictates what can and cannot be accomplished or enjoyed on any given day.

But what if you could outwit or overpower your captor? Suppose, like a prisoner of war, you are obliged to devise a way of escape instead of waiting for an unlikely truce? What would you call yourself if you succeeded in overcoming the limitations imposed by arthritis?

Enter the Hero

You can and should take charge of the management of your health and your life. First—and possibly most important—you've got to rid yourself of the "victim mentality." Despite arthritis, it's important for you to wring some joy and satisfaction from your daily life. Both your mental and physical health will benefit.

Once free from that feeling of powerlessness, you can plan a program to help you regain strength and mobility. It will include good nutrition and sensible exercise, along with natural (nondrug) treatments such as massage and hydrotherapy. It also will include ways to handle pain—ways that free you from taking drugs to dull your senses, or drugs with dangerous side effects.

As you read the remainder of this book, you'll discover that regardless of what form of arthritis you have, a variety of therapies are available. Review all the options open to you, and weigh the benefits and drawbacks of each. Devise your own plan to manage not only the symptoms of arthritis but the quality of your life.

6

THE SPUNK FACTOR

*There is nothing either good or bad but thinking
makes it so.*

Hamlet, *William Shakespeare*

In some ways, the most difficult problem with having arthritis lies not in the joints but in the mind. And that problem can grow as the years add up.

Listen to this tale of two arthritics. Mary J., a plump, merry woman in her early 50s, was diagnosed as having arthritis in her knees. Her doctor strongly suggested that she lose 50 or 60 pounds and take up a mild exercise such as swimming—not only to help her shed weight but also to keep the muscles, tendons, and ligaments around her joints strong and healthy.

Mary worked as an advertising copywriter in midtown Manhattan, spending most of her day sitting at a desk. She liked lunching in some of New York's gourmet eateries, and was not inspired to diet. Moreover, she felt "too old, too fat, and too sick" to take up swimming. Her major exercise, in fact, was climbing two long flights of stairs to and from the subway platform. It was this climb that caused Mary the worst pain of the day.

One morning, as Mary slowly eased her heavy frame down the subway steps, a young man in a hurry bumped into her so that she lost her precarious balance and pitched forward down the stairs. She fell, skinning the heel of her hand and one knee.

Mary was very angry with the young man, but she was even angrier at her body, and its inability to function the way it always used to. When she arrived at the office, she called her husband. "I've had it with the subway. I don't feel well and I really can't make the trip to and from work anymore. I'd like to take a sick leave, or maybe even resign," she said.

At about the same time, across the East River in Queens, Helen G. was listening to her doctor explain what to expect now that she had been diagnosed as having osteoarthritis.

An attractive housewife in her late 40s, Helen did not feel upset by the diagnosis. "I'd been sick before with things like colds and the flu. During college I had a long, painful bout with mono. But I always pulled through, just as good as new. So I figured I'd just keep active, do what the doctor tells me, and I'll be able to handle this problem."

As the years passed, the difference in the attitudes of these two women had a major effect on the quality of their lives.

Mary felt limited by her pain and depressed because each morning it was still there to greet her. She quit her job and withdrew to her bedroom, where she watched television and napped. She considered herself an invalid, and indeed, became one.

Helen, on the other hand, rode out the worst episodes of pain. Buoyed by even the slightest improvement, she would test herself by setting tasks that were within the realm of accomplishment. She walked her dog, sat out in the sun, volunteered to help at the church's craft bazaar, and joined a group that discussed best-selling books. While her life was not exactly the same as before she developed arthritis, it was good enough. There were many moments of satisfaction, accomplishment, and even joy.

Steve Pickert, M.D., a family practitioner in Thurmont, Maryland, has treated many patients with arthritis. He says, "People who get depressed get worse faster. Others who maintain a positive attitude can work with the disease. A lot depends on your *perception* of pain. Your emotional reaction

to chronic illness will not make your arthritis worse—but it
will make your life worse. You have to make the most of what
you have. You can live an almost normal life with all but the
most severe forms of arthritis.

"I give my patients a pep talk. I can see in their faces
whether they're feeling depressed or not. I know the disease
is cyclical and that if they can get through the slump they'll
be feeling better again. So I try to give them encouragement,
particularly about keeping active and involved."

Indeed, activity and involvement are of primary importance. For one thing, when you are actively involved in
something you enjoy—whether it's jogging or jigsaw
puzzles—your mind is distracted from pain. In his book *Free
Yourself from Pain* (Simon and Schuster, 1979), author David
E. Bresler, Ph.D., describes the progress of a woman called
Peggy, whose life has been devastated by blinding headaches.
Peggy keeps a daily log that correlates her activities with the
degree of pain she feels. In it she notes that during a phone
call from her daughter she was "barely aware of discomfort,"
and that, while planning with her husband for a summer
vacation, she felt "maybe there is still room for pleasure in
my life."

In addition to relief from pain and depression, involvement in a pleasurable activity promotes a sense of accomplishment and self-worth. Dr. Bresler, who is the director of
the Bresler Center for Allied Therapeutics in Los Angeles,
California, as well as an author, says, "People with chronic
pain often don't do things they would normally enjoy. They
feel they can't because of the pain. But it's often the other
way around. Their pain actually persists longer because they
don't have any fun." In fact, Dr. Bresler routinely inquires
about his patients' "serum fun levels," an important indicator of a person's well-being.

Sure, it isn't easy to push yourself when you're hurting
and there's no relief in sight. However, psychologists have
developed a number of techniques that can help you change
the way you perceive what's happening to you, so that you
feel more positive and optimistic, and consequently, feel
better physically. One such psychologist is Gary Emery,
Ph.D., an assistant clinical professor at the University of

California at Los Angeles and director of the Los Angeles Center for Cognitive Therapy. Dr. Emery says, "When you're depressed you think nothing will help you, and so you don't try to help yourself. Your threshold to pain is lower. You want to hide out or sleep. But people who force themselves to take action against depression will come out of it."

Motivation Follows Action

Dr. Emery has devised an action-packed program to lift you out of depression. His plan is based on a treatment approach called cognitive therapy, an approach that says it's the way you *think* about your experiences that determines how you react to them. Some erroneous thinking may fool you into believing there are a lot of things you can't do—that you really can.

The first step, he says, is to correct your thinking errors about having arthritis. Write down your thoughts or use a tape recorder to express your feelings about having the disease. Then, review what you have said, looking for these common errors in thinking:

1. *Exaggerating.* Just how bad is your arthritis pain? Is it *really* as bad as you just said? Rate it on a scale of 0 to 100 to see if you are exaggerating.

2. *Jumping to conclusions.* By jumping to conclusions you can make wrong assumptions. An example of jumping to conclusions would be, "Some arthritis treatments may help others but they probably won't work for me" and "I can't go to the store because my arthritis is too bad today."

3. *Ignoring rescue or safety factors.* With this thinking error, you focus on just the worst aspect of the disease, ignoring things that can help or even facets of life that remain unaffected by the disease.

4. *Overgeneralizing.* With this error, you're likely to say that if one joint hurts, then everything is (or soon will be) terrible. People who say, "I have ar-

thritis, I'm getting old, I guess I'm worthless," are guilty of this kind of thinking.

5. *Catastrophizing.* Here, a person will say, "I've got arthritis. I'm going to be crippled. I'll be at the mercy of others."

Suppose you do make some (or even all) of these errors in thinking. What should you do? According to Dr. Emery, you begin to change your thinking by first accepting the fact that you have arthritis. Then, start building toward a new set of beliefs.

Once you are aware of your self-defeating thoughts, answer them with more realistic perceptions. Without exaggeration or overgeneralization, you can cut your emotional reaction to having arthritis right down to size.

Finally, take action. "*Don't* talk to everybody about your arthritis. Don't make it a big deal in your own mind, or to others. Complaining about the pain keeps your mind focused on it," suggests Dr. Emery. "*Do* make a list of diversions— things like talking on the phone, reading, working at a hobby or craft. When you begin to feel bad, try to divert your attention from the pain by working on one of the diversions from your list," he says.

Or, take a challenge action. "Try to go to the store, and see what happens," he says. Once the depression lifts, Dr. Emery says, you will not be as bothered by the pain. "Depressed, you personalize the pain as though no one else in the world ever had pain. But keep in mind that most of the work of the world is done by people who don't feel very well," he says.

Action and Reaction

What kinds of activities can you undertake? Any you think will give you enjoyment. If your arthritis isn't too severe, a strenuous exercise program—first approved by your doctor—may be just the ticket. If exercise seems too difficult, try something satisfying but less strenuous. Even a quiet hobby like needlepoint or knitting can have very real benefits.

Why should activities as diverse as stretching and stitching help free you from pain? Certainly, as Dr. Emery suggests, your mind becomes diverted from thinking about pain. But more is involved.

A quiet activity like knitting can trigger a "relaxation response." According to Herbert Benson, M.D., author of *The Mind/Body Effect* (Simon and Schuster, 1979), a lot of people feel relaxed while doing handwork because the activity is so similar to meditation. And that sort of profound relaxation can cause the brain to release marvelous, natural painkillers called endorphins. Exercise, too, causes the brain to release the same chemicals. According to Charles W. Denko, M.D., Ph.D., preliminary findings show that on days when arthritis patients feel good about life, they have higher levels of endorphins in their blood.

He and his colleagues have studied the relationship between arthritis and endorphins at George Scott Research Laboratories, Fairview General Hospital, Cleveland, Ohio. Dr. Denko found that arthritis patients usually have lower levels of endorphins than healthy people. Moreover, the patients who complained of extreme pain—for example, some gout patients—had almost no endorphins in their synovial fluid and extremely low levels in their blood. But when the patients reported feeling chipper, sure enough, their endorphin level was higher.

Now which came first—the upbeat mood or the up-level of endorphins? There is some evidence that the mind can control levels of these natural painkillers. In fact, this theory may explain how the placebo effect works.

Placebos—usually a harmless, nonmedicinal substance—somehow manage to help people every day. The effect is so common it must be considered in every scientific test involving people. Here's how it works. Give a group of patients some fake pills or a harmless saltwater injection and tell them they're receiving a powerful drug that will make them feel better. Sure enough, a certain percent (usually about a third) will feel better. What's important, apparently, is not the treatment itself but the patient's *belief* in its effectiveness.

Endorphins appear to play a key role in this remarkable

occurrence. In one study at the University of California at San Francisco, 23 dental patients who had teeth pulled a few hours earlier were injected with a placebo. A third reported that their pain eased up as a result. But when they were injected with a second substance that blocked the action of the endorphins, pain returned to all of them. Apparently, their belief that the placebo was working triggered the release of those natural painkillers.

Wouldn't it be wonderful if we could just take two placebo pills every time our joints are jumping? Of course we can't, but that doesn't mean we can't use the painkilling power in our bodies. As we said, exercise, relaxation, even the *belief* in our ability to be pain-free, will do the trick. But there's another way, too. A new way that allows you to "see" your pain, and, perhaps, see it on its way out.

The technique is called pain-control imagery. With it, the pain sufferer talks to his body and its source of pain, eventually establishing an open dialogue with it, and thereby a means of control. In his book *Free Yourself from Pain,* Dr. Bresler describes how the technique worked for one patient.

John, a 52-year-old cardiologist, lived with constant, agonizing, low-back pain following treatment for rectal cancer. The pain, he said, was "unbearable," and had reduced his options to three: successful treatment, somewhere; voluntary commitment to a mental institution; or suicide. He could not go on living without relief. In desperation, he sought the help of a psychologist at the pain-control unit of a local hospital.

In reviewing John's records, the psychologist noticed that during an earlier psychiatric workup, John had described his pain with terrible vividness: It was like "a dog chewing on my spine," he had said. Believing that this image was more than merely picturesque—that it was, in fact, a sort of nightmarish picture postcard from the source of his pain—the psychologist tried to convince John to make contact with the dog, talk to it to find out why it was chewing his spine, and somehow make it stop.

With his training in traditional medicine, John at first considered the idea absurd, but his pain was so intense that he decided to give it a try. Over a series of sessions, the psychologist taught John to relax physically and mentally, and open his mind to the image of the dog. Then John started talking to it—and the dog talked back.

The dog said John never really wanted to be a doctor in the first place; he'd wanted to be an architect, but his mother had pressured him into medical school. As a result, his smoldering resentment was directed at his mother, his colleagues, and his patients. It was also directed inward, the dog said, and had contributed to the development of his cancer and his low-back pain, too.

The dog told John he was a good doctor. "It may not be the career you wanted," he said, "but it's time you recognized how good you are at what you do. When you stop being so resentful and start accepting yourself, I'll stop chewing on your spine." These insights were accompanied by an immediate easing of the pain, and during the following weeks, it slowly subsided.

It may sound like an unorthodox—not to say just plain nutty—approach to the problem of chronic pain. "After all, what would be your initial reaction to a doctor who encouraged you to talk to little animals in your head?" asks Dr. Bresler.

Nutty or not, for many who are wary of taking painkillers for years on end, or who have tried standard therapies and found them lacking, a technique like pain-control imagery could provide blessed relief.

By "talking" to our bodies, we can learn to control endorphin release. Dr. Bresler explains that this inner dialogue also contacts the autonomic nervous system, which controls such involuntary functions as heart rate and digestion, and plays a critical role in the relief of chronic pain.

Because the autonomic nervous system is linked to the unconscious part of our minds—the part that processes information in an abstract, symbolic way—the only language it understands is symbolism and imagery. We can reach parts of our bodies controlled by the conscious mind with verbal commands: "Fingers, turn the page of this book," or "Foot, slide into the shoe." But to the unconscious mind, these commands are a foreign language. To talk to it, Dr. Bresler says, we need a new language, though "the land of imagery is largely neglected, and its language is often as unfamiliar as one spoken in a faraway country."

For example, try telling your mouth to "produce and secrete saliva" (an involuntary function). Any luck? Then try—as clearly and as vividly as possible—imagining a fresh, juicy, yellow lemon. Imagine the spray of bright, tart juice as you slice it open with a knife. Then, take a wet slice and slip it into your mouth, tasting its incredible sourness, its sharpness, its wetness. Did that work any better?

With practice and guidance, the power of this kind of mental image-making can be harnessed to ease pain caused by everything from arthritis to angina. And in pain-control centers around the country, the use of imagery techniques has become increasingly common.

In essence, imagery techniques are a way of reestablishing contact between mind and body. How Western medicine ever separated the two in the first place is a long story, but what is now becoming abundantly clear is that they've had a marvelously complex and intimate affair going all along, like two lovers conversing with winks and signals across a crowded room. Each one, it's now known, has an astonishing degree of control over the other. The end result of this relationship can be remarkable occurrences like the placebo effect, or anesthesia as the result of hypnosis or acupuncture.

The exact techniques used for the control of pain will be described later in the book. Right now, it's important for you, or anyone with arthritis, to understand that pain can be controlled—and controlled without using dangerous drugs. Even more important is the understanding that any person can take responsibility for his or her own health. Instead of waiting for the doctor to devise some new treatment, it's important for you to exert some control over your own life. By staying involved, by caring about things outside of the self, by believing that you can overcome, you will overcome.

7

PREVENTION IS POSSIBLE: ARTHRITIS ISN'T INEVITABLE

Taking charge of your life and your health can begin quite early. In fact, the very first measure you can take against arthritis is prevention.

"Most kinds of arthritis are easy to prevent if you pay attention to diet, supplements, exercise, and any allergies you may have," says Ray Wunderlich, M.D., who specializes in preventive medicine in his St. Petersburg, Florida, practice.

Earlier in this book we explained that many forms of arthritis are hereditary. It would seem, then, that they are inevitable. However, such is not the case. Your genes can give you an inherited flaw or weakness that makes you susceptible to getting the disease under certain circumstances. But suppose you could avoid those circumstances, or compensate for them in some way. Chances are you could prevent arthritis or delay it for a very long time. And that, really, is what Dr. Wunderlich advises his patients. His techniques for avoiding those elements in life called "precipitating factors"—that is, those situations that can bring about the disease—involve maintaining a scrupulously healthy lifestyle.

Preventive Exercise

The first and foremost weapon in his preventive arsenal is exercise. "We don't grow old and stiff, but stiff and old," the doctor likes to say. Sure enough, there are several medical studies that support Dr. Wunderlich's theory that exercise can prevent arthritis. One of the first studies attempted to find just how much damage to the joints is caused by strenuous exercise. It involved studying the hip joints of 74 former Finnish runners, with an average age of 55, most of whom had raced for more than 20 years.

Surprise! Instead of finding *more* osteoarthritis in these runners, researchers at the Oulu University Central Hospital in Finland found *less*. Only 4 percent of the athletes had developed osteoarthritis. The study concluded that competitive sports cannot be considered as a factor that makes osteoarthritis more likely. It said, "Anatomically and physiologically, it is not strange that the hips of competitive runners should be spared osteoarthritis, for the hip is designed for walking and running, and motion is necessary for the nutrition of the cartilage."

Indeed, joints need to move in order to breathe—not air, but the special synovial fluid required to lubricate and feed the joints. An orthopedic surgeon writing in the *British Medical Journal* describes this "feeding" as a process of "intermittent compression and release" by which synovial fluid enters and leaves the cartilage "in very much the same way as air enters and leaves the lungs." What happens when we lie idle for too long, the surgeon warns, is that cartilage begins to run dry. Immobilization for only six days "produces ulceration and destruction of the cartilage."

In another study, this done by the Rheumatism Research Unit of the General Infirmary at Leeds, Great Britain, X rays of the hips and knees of 364 women were examined for signs of osteoarthritis. These women were chosen for study because they were teachers of physical education, and considered a likely group to have developed osteoarthritis as a result of the daily physical pounding their joints received. Surprise again! While moderate to severe osteoarthritis was as common in the teachers as it was in the general population, there were *significantly* fewer cases of mild osteoarthritis.

According to George Ehrlich, M.D., director of the Arthritis Center at Philadelphia's Albert Einstein Medical Center, the reason exercise works—in addition to feeding the joint cartilage—is that "by strengthening the muscles around the joint, exercise makes the joint work better." Stronger muscles mean less wear and tear on cartilage and bone, and less chance of deterioration or osteoarthritis.

A WORD OF CAUTION

More important than the kind of exercise you do is the *way* you do it. If you exercise improperly, in fact, you can hasten the development of the disease. In particular, avoid exercising without a thorough warm-up; when muscles are tight, the joint moves unnaturally, producing damaging strains.

The second important aspect of exercising is to do it at least three or four times a week for at least 20 minutes a session. A sweaty hour of calisthenics once a week simply doesn't cut it, but daily, repetitious activities—like walking or swimming—are superb. How about running and jogging? They're fine, provided you use common sense. Run on a good, smooth surface that "gives," wear good shoes, and pay scrupulous attention to warm-up exercises and stretching.

Dr. Wunderlich also cautions that you should not depend entirely on activities that use only one side of the body, such as racquetball or bowling. Overuse of just one side can create an imbalance in the body and consequently stress the joints. Instead, he recommends supplementing sports like these with a good general exercise, such as swimming, aerobic dancing, trampolining on a rebounder, or running. "It gets your heart going," he says, "and you need a good pump to circulate nutrition to your cells." He also suggests doing exercises just for the joints—exercises that stretch. These include acrobatics, dancing, yoga, aerobic dancing, and even belly dancing. (Good for the spine, for sure!)

"It's never too late to begin a program of prevention," says Dr. Wunderlich. "At 40, 50, or 60, you've still got a good chance. But remember that the older you get, the greater the risk. Accumulated errors of living finally come out in the body's most susceptible area. So exercise. Gradualism is the key in building the body. Too much, too soon leads to injury and discouragement. Better to go slow and enjoy the improvement! Remember the joints are made to move."

Avoiding Injuries

Another important step in prevention is avoiding injuries that can result in the disease. Now, while we can hardly cancel all future accidents and falls, by their very nature unplanned, we can avoid many of the little injuries we inflict upon ourselves each day. Tight shoes are a good example. Not only do they cause pain, they also can cause arthritis in the toe joints. Using some common sense, you can avoid a crippling problem in the future. Purchase shoes for fit rather than fashion. Make sure your toes do not butt against the front of the shoe, and that they have enough room to wiggle and spread.

If you work at a job that keeps you on your feet a lot, it might pay to install a sponge rubber mat in front of your work area—whether it's a machine, blackboard, or kitchen sink.

We know that certain occupations seem to set up conditions for the development of specific kinds of arthritis. For example, if you work for many years as a typist you are more likely to develop arthritis in the neck than any other place. Likewise, pneumatic drill operators get it in their wrists, coal miners get it in their elbows, and gamblers who play slot machines develop it in their right shoulder.

What to do to prevent the "inevitable"?

USE A GOOD CHAIR

It's estimated that 75 percent of us have to sit while we earn our living. Since we spend the better part of the day on our bottoms, let's take a hard look at what this position does to us.

Did you know that sitting can produce more pressure on spinal disks than standing? And in a slumped sitting position, vertebrae of the lower back are tipped exhaustingly forward, a condition that can produce as much ligament strain at the base of the spine as heavy lifting. But that's not all sitting can do.

The arrangement of the body in various chairs can affect a wide range of muscles and nerves and interfere with the functioning of vital organs.

Is your chair positioning you for future arthritis? Stand up and find out. Some elaborate tests have determined the following features to be well worth looking for in a chair.

First, the Seat Portion

• It should have a rounded front. Too sharp an edge can restrict blood flow to the underpart of the thighs, causing numbness and tingling.

• It should be adjustable in height, and adjusted so that your feet come into firm—but not too firm—contact with the floor. A seat that's too high can cause feet to dangle, thus increasing pressure on the underpart of the thighs; and one that's too low can force you to sit in a jackknifed position, putting undue strain on the lower back as it is obliged to curl.

• It should not be soft so you can't squirm around. Studies have shown that sitters like to move around periodically. It's the body's way of preventing muscle spasms and aiding blood flow, and a seat cushion that's too soft makes such movement difficult.

Next, the Backrest

• It should come only about a third of the way up the back. If it's a recliner, be sure it has a headrest.

• Just above the surface of the seat, there should be either an open space or an area indented enough to allow the buttocks to get moved slightly to the rear of the lower back. Above this open area (which is also good for allowing air circulation and shirttail room), there should be a slight protrusion to encourage the back to be held in a slightly forward arch.

• And for rest periods, a chair that inclines may be a good idea. Movement back and forth from an upright position to an inclined one also helps transport nutrients to disks between the vertebrae.

A KIND OF BED SORE

Aside from your chair, the other piece of furniture you spend a lot of time on is your bed. A good mattress is very important in keeping the spine, back muscles, and ligaments free of strain. Since you spend a third of your life in bed, the quality of your resting spot, or lack of it, can have a lot to do with the future health of your spine and hips.

Doctors recognize the problems a wrong bed can create, but they can't agree on a solution. Probably because there isn't one. There are many.

"No bed is perfectly suited for everyone," says Robert G. Addison, M.D., associate professor of orthopedic surgery at Northwestern University Medical School in Chicago, Illinois. He should know because he has helped design mattresses for major bedding manufacturers. "However, the ideal mattress should cradle the spine in the same position as if you were standing with good posture," he says.

Usually that takes a firm mattress. Our body weight is not evenly distributed, so we need adequate support under places that sink deepest into the mattress—the hips, chest, and head in particular. A good mattress should distribute weight evenly so that one part of the body is not stressed more than another.

"In designing a mattress, we use a system called angles of deflection according to body weight," explains Dr. Addison. "That means we measure how much the mattress dips when pressures from the head, shoulders, hips, and feet are exerted on it. In a well-constructed mattress, these angles of deflection should vary less than 5 percent. This indicates that the person's weight is very evenly distributed—exactly what a good mattress should do."

But not all mattresses are created equal, and consequently, some do not distribute body weight in the most desirable way.

To prove that point and to find out which beds did the job best, an experiment was conducted. "Of course we couldn't test every bed on the market," said Steven Garfin, M.D., of the University of California at San Diego. "But we did test four of them—an 'orthopedic' hard bed containing 720 coils in the mattress plus a bed board and box spring, a standard 500-coil soft bed, a standard 10-inch-deep water bed, and a new hybrid bed composed of a central core of water surrounded by polyurethane foam."

Five volunteers (all in good health) were asked to lie on each of the beds, which had first been covered with a special pressure-measuring sheet.

What the researchers found, says Dr. Garfin, was that in both the prone (on the stomach) and supine (on the back) positions, the hard bed and the water bed distributed weight more evenly over the entire body than the other beds. The soft bed and the hybrid bed, on the other hand, recorded extremely uneven pressures. In fact, all five persons studied felt the latter two beds were uncomfortable, while there were no complaints about the other two.

Shortly after the study was completed, Dr. Garfin decided to test the same four beds again, only this time all the volunteers chosen suffered from chronic low-back pain.

"The standard 'orthopedic' bed that is hard or extra firm is generally the type of bed recommended by most physicians and textbooks dealing with chronic low-back pain," explains Dr. Garfin.

"Water beds are, in fact, discouraged by most doctors who treat this condition. But then we'll meet people with chronic low-back pain and they'll tell us that water beds work for them.

"Presumably, firm mattresses are effective in relieving back pain by helping straighten the lumbar (lower) back," explains Dr. Garfin. "But, if that's true, a water bed theoretically should not afford any relief. Weight distribution on a water bed is even and the spinal contours are probably unchanged. Yet, one half of the patients in this study felt symptomatic relief on this bed. As expected, the other half listed the hard bed as their first choice.

"Of interest," adds Dr. Garfin, "was that all patients

except one felt that the hybrid bed caused a deterioration in their condition, and in fact, two patients quit the study early after sleeping on the hybrid bed.

"When it comes to low-back pain," Dr. Garfin told us, "a hard bed is still the preferred support structure. However, a water bed offers an alternative to those patients not helped by the hard bed."

But choosing a bed for comfort alone is not always a wise move.

Lionel A. Walpin, M.D., who is clinical director of physical medicine and rehabilitation at Cedars-Sinai Medical Center in Los Angeles, California, says, "Sleep is our longest single postural activity and we have the least control of it." For those who experience pain or stiffness on arising, Dr. Walpin explains there are two major kinds.

"Postural pain comes on gradually. You may notice it developing after hunching over a desk for an hour or so. It's relieved, however, when you stand up and stretch, or just change your position. A person with pure postural pain is the one who has full mobility but who wakes up in the morning stiff and sore. He was probably sleeping in wrong positions for hours, but because the pain came on slowly it didn't cause him to wake during the night. This person can choose a mattress for comfort alone and that should relieve his postural distress."

PRODDING THE SPINE INTO SHAPE

"With dysfunctional pain, on the other hand, you wake up suddenly during the night with pain, but on awakening in the morning you can feel fine," Dr. Walpin adds. "Then you stand up, bend over and—wham—instant pain again. With dysfunction (abnormal function of muscles and joints), you don't have full mobility. Also, treating only the pain, in this case, is not synonymous with recovery. You need to restore the normal strength, length, and flexibility of the dysfunctioning muscles and joints, too.

"Choosing a bed for comfort alone would probably be a mistake here because it may foster the continuation of the problem. People with dysfunctional pain need a firm mattress. But I have patients who will tell me that they were sleeping on a soft bed, bought a firm one, and now their backs hurt more than ever. That's because a firm mattress tries to put you in the proper position by restoring the normal curvatures of your spine. The muscles and ligaments are being stretched and balanced (which is good), but, at first, this can also hurt.

"On the other hand," says Dr. Walpin, "if you continue to sleep on a soft bed, you wind up continuing to have unbalanced muscles that are too short on one side of the spine and too stretched on the other. At first, it may actually feel better to you than the firm mattress only because you are compensating for these abnormal, weak muscles—the very ones you are trying to correct. But, because the dysfunction continues, you remain more susceptible to physical stress and strain and a worsening of the very condition you're trying to cure."

Naturally, we can't recommend a particular brand of bed for you. We can't even say for certain that an inner-spring mattress is definitely better than a water bed, or that an air or foam mattress won't work as well. But we can give you some guidelines. Dr. Walpin believes that "versatility in all bedding products is the ideal." For instance, he helped develop a unique bed pillow that is named for him and that offers four different degrees of head and neck support simply by turning the pillow around or over.

And, before you buy a new bed, you may want to improve the one you've already got. "You can customize your own bed board," suggests Dr. Walpin. "Instead of using a solid piece of plywood under your mattress, cut individual wood slats to fit your bed. Make each slat about 4 feet by 1½ feet. Then you can move the slats to where you need the most support."

If that doesn't help enough, you can start shopping. But don't be hasty. This is one purchase that deserves your time and attention. A five-second flop on a couple of beds in the local mattress store just will not do.

"If you have to try out a mattress in the store," advises Dr. Addison, "lie down on it for ten minutes at least. Study what happens to the bed as you vary your position. When you lie on your back, your buttocks should be supported and you should feel that support. You should be able to lie comfortably on your stomach without unnaturally arching your back, although I don't recommend this as a primary sleeping position. On your side, your shoulders and hips should sink in slightly so that your spine settles into a horizontal, not a curved position."

And remember, when it comes to firmness, don't be swayed by manufacturers' labels such as super-firm, ultra-firm, or the very medical-sounding ortho-firm. There are no industry-wide standards when it comes to bedding descriptions, so what you feel is what you get.

What you get you may have to take lying down, so to speak, for years to come.

Overloading Weight-Bearing Supports

Finally, a word about fat. The weight-bearing joints—primarily the hips and knees, but also the ankles—are perfectly capable of carrying the weight of an adult body. However, many people with arthritis in their knees or hips are overweight. These joints were not meant to heft around an extra 50 or 100 pounds, 365 days a year. The strain can destroy the joint. Moreover, the tendons and ligaments can become separated by the thick layer of fat, so the joints no longer are mechanically correct. Again, strain is the result. Finally, if you are fat, chances are the fat levels in your blood—that's cholesterol and triglycerides—are higher than they should be. Some doctors have found in their practices that people with these high fat levels in their blood tend to develop certain kinds of arthritis.

If you can pinch more than an inch of flesh at your beltline, you should diet. Try to achieve the weight you were when you were 20.

* * *

While all this information may seem terribly ordinary, things you knew all along—exercise, avoid injuries, eat right, don't get fat—it represents a ray of hope for many. If your grandparents and parents have arthritis, it does not mean that you are destined to have it, too. And if you already have developed the disease, this advice offers a program that can help spare your children or your younger sisters and brothers.

Each and every day, medical science comes upon yet another discovery that shows our bodies were meant to work hard and function well. It seems that if we give our physical selves a fighting chance by removing obstacles that result from an unhealthy lifestyle, our bodies will reward us by staying strong and fit.

8

AFFIRMATIVE ACTION THROUGH NUTRITION

Ah, the things others take for granted: stuffing a turkey and nestling it into a roasting pan, carrying a tureen of homemade soup to the table, triumphantly lugging baskets of vegetables fresh from the garden, kneading a batch of silky bread dough. For many people with arthritis, these tasks may be possible only on special days—days when the pain lets up and the swelling goes down. And for some, they're only memories.

Good eating may also be a memory. Because food shopping and preparation can be difficult, those with arthritis sometimes are unable to fill their basic nutritional needs. Many rely on processed foods—TV dinners, instant potatoes, canned meat and pasta combinations, cookies, soup mix, and the like. Others live on tea and toast, gradually wasting away to frailty. In fact, aside from joint pain, the one thing many people with arthritis may have in common is poor nutrition.

Unfortunately, even for those who do manage to eat well-balanced, nourishing meals, there's still a catch. Because of physical limitations, they often do not exercise sufficiently. As a result, the pounds pile on, putting great strain on the weight-bearing joints.

A chronic illness like arthritis, in some very subtle and unsuspected ways, can lead to other health problems unless diet is closely watched. These problems include high blood pressure, obesity, heart disease, stroke, and diabetes. At the risk of stating the obvious, good nutrition is necessary for good health. To outlast arthritis, stay involved with life, find some pleasure in each day, and avoid potential health complications, it's of paramount importance to eat right. Even if you do hurt. Moreover, people with arthritis may have special dietary requirements that help them fight off the worst of the disease. These will be discussed separately in the next chapter.

What happens when you turn to the can opener or the foil-wrapped frozen slab for dinner is that you end the problem of meal preparation but begin developing some real dietary problems. When we rely on food prepared by others (particularly others who hope to turn a tidy profit on it), we often get more—and less—than we bargained for. We get more salt, sugar, and calories; less honest-to-goodness nutrition.

Salt: Seen and Hidden

Let's begin by examining the hidden salt content in just a few common processed foods. Take peas, for example. A ½-cup serving of fresh peas has only 2 milligrams of salt. But the same size serving of frozen peas contains 92 milligrams, and ½ cup of canned peas hides a whopping 200 milligrams of salt. Pea soup? Have a tiny ½-cup serving and the sodium tab hits 450 milligrams.

At least the flavor of these products hints at the salt content, although most people would never guess the high amount. But some products with a very sweet—not salty—flavor also contain substantial quantities of sodium. These are really sneaky. For instance, a 12-ounce bottle of Pepsi has anywhere from 35 to 49 milligrams of salt. The sweetness in a serving of carrots with brown sugar glaze hides an impressive 500 milligrams of salt.

So processed foods contain a lot of salt. What's the big deal about eating a little salt, you may ask. First, it's not just a *little* salt. Americans consume 10 to 15 times the amount our bodies need. Health professionals believe that the high salt content in our diet may be an important factor in the development of hypertension (high blood pressure), which affects about 35 million Americans and contributes to several hundred thousand deaths from heart attacks and strokes every year.

Why does excessive salt cause your pressure to go up? There's an old saying, "Water goes where the salt is." Because sodium clings to water, when an excessive amount enters the cellular fluid, it carries extra water with it. This extra liquid increases the volume of the plasma. In order to distribute the expanded blood, the heart must create additional pressure and therefore pump harder.

Excessive salt intake may also trigger migraine headaches. In one study, 10 out of 12 patients with proven migraines had lower incidences of recurrent headaches after restricting salt intake from snack foods on an empty stomach.

Some people believe that sea salt may be an acceptable substitute for table salt. Others worry that if they do not consume salt, they may not be getting enough iodine, thus running the risk of developing a goiter. While we're on the topic of salt, let's put those two myths to rest.

The only real difference between sea salt and regular salt is the price. Sea salt costs up to four times more than regular table salt. Many people are willing to pay that price because they believe the product contains extra nutrients. Sea salt *would* be rich in minerals if it were just evaporated sea water, which has large amounts of magnesium, calcium, and potassium. But it isn't.

Sea salt is purified to meet government standards which require that all "food-grade" salt, whether taken from the sea or from salt mines, be at least 97.5 percent sodium chloride—salt. That doesn't leave much room for other minerals. For all practical purposes, sea salt and regular salt are just about the same. So if you come across an "all natural" product that lists sea salt on the label, avoid it just as you would any product containing salt.

And for those who worry about goiter, take heart. A lack of iodine in the diet (and the result of this deficiency, goiter) was only a problem in the days when people ate fruits and vegetables grown in iodine-poor soil and couldn't get produce from anywhere else. Health officials introduced iodized salt during the 1920s as a way of dealing with this problem. Today, however, produce grown in iodine-rich soils is available all over the country. In addition, fish—which has lots of iodine—is also available everywhere.

If you're really worried about goiter, don't continue using salt. Instead, turn to kelp. A teaspoon a day will provide you with more than 20 times the Recommended Dietary Allowance for iodine.

Fiber: Among the Missing

When manufacturers package food, they aim to please the common palate. Salty flavor is okay, but heaviness or chewiness is not. You'll notice that in the box of macaroni and cheese, for example, the macaroni is always white—never whole wheat. A roll of unbaked biscuit dough, likewise, is white. Canned and frozen vegetables are always peeled. Boxed cereal may be "fortified" with vitamins and iron, but the grains they're made from have been stripped of their bran.

What's the end result of all this processing? For one thing, the food lacks fiber. In just the past few years, there's been an explosion of information about the importance of this dietary element. It's been found that fiber can prevent constipation and thus reduce the risk of hemorrhoids, diverticular disease of the colon, hiatus hernia, and varicose veins.

Moreover, it's been found that diets loaded with fiber can protect against cancer of the colon (and other diet-related cancers), help prevent or treat diabetes, work against the formation of gallstones, lower high blood pressure, and even keep you from getting fat.

Most people tend to think of fiber as just one substance. Actually, it's many, ranging from the pectin found in fruit to gums and celluloses. All forms of fiber are totally free of calories but nevertheless very filling because of their bulk.

The world expert on fiber, Denis P. Burkitt, recommends that you not rely on just bran to provide that "roughage." You need all the varieties available in fresh, whole foods because it is the *combination* of celluloses, pentoses, pectin, gums, and lignin that does the trick.

Ten foods high in fiber are spinach, corn, peas, blackberries, sweet potatoes, apples, whole wheat bread, potatoes, broccoli, and zucchini.

Sugar: How Sweet It Is

Another significant problem in relying too heavily on "convenience foods" is that they contain too much sugar. And, again, it's hidden in the product. Even the United States Department of Agriculture has admitted that sugar is getting harder and harder to avoid because 75 percent of what we use is nondiscretionary. That's a fancy way of saying that we have no control over the total amount we consume each day because fully 75 percent of what we eat has been added to processed or take-out food by the manufacturers or retailers. Sugar is added to such seemingly innocuous foods as ketchup, peanut butter, and breakfast cereal, possibly accounting for the big jump in sugar consumption in this country—up from 104 to 126 pounds per year in the last 61 years. That's eating almost your own weight in sugar each year!

We all would be wise to control our sugar consumption because this simple carbohydrate provides nothing but calories. It offers *no* nutrition. Moreover, it tends to deplete the thiamine in our bodies, can lead to or aggravate both hypoglycemia and diabetes, can promote tooth decay, and has even been shown to depress the immune response, which means we have lowered resistance to disease. Add to this the relatively unknown medical fact that sugar can also combine in a special way with salt to promote high blood pressure, and it's easy to see that sugar is not just a harmless sweet.

Certainly we can monitor some of our sugar consumption. Should someone ask, "One lump or two?" we have the opportunity to decide on just one, or better yet, none. But when the sugar has been added to our food before we even purchase it, gauging how much we eat becomes a more difficult task. The trick is to read labels very carefully.

Food manufacturers are required to list the ingredients in a product according to their quantity. Thus, if the primary ingredient in a food is wheat, it is listed first on the label, with the remaining ingredients listed in their descending order. It would seem easy to spot sugar if the manufacturer obeys labeling regulations. However, food manufacturers often use more than one name for sugar to obscure its high percentage in a product. They may list it as sucrose, dextrose, corn

Table 4: **SELECTED DIETARY SOURCES OF FIBER**

Food	Serving Size	Total Fiber (grams)	Food	Serving Size	Total Fiber (grams)
Spinach, cooked	1 cup	11.4	Pinto beans	½ cup	3.1
Corn	1 cup	7.8	Strawberries	1 cup	3.1
Peas, raw	1 cup	7.6	Beets	1 cup	3.0
Blackberries	1 cup	7.4	Peanuts	¼ cup	3.0
Sweet potato	1 medium	7.2	Orange	1 medium	2.9
Apple	1 medium	6.8	Kale, cooked	1 cup	2.8
Whole wheat bread	2 slices	5.4	Rolled oats	1 cup	2.8
Potato	1 medium	5.3	Coconut	¼ cup	2.7
Broccoli, cooked	1 cup	5.2	Apricots	4 medium	2.6
Almonds	¼ cup	5.1	Brown rice	1 cup	2.6
Raisins	½ cup	5.0	Asparagus	1 cup	2.4
Zucchini	1 cup	5.0	Celery	2 stalks	2.4
Plums	4 medium	4.6	Barley	½ cup	2.2
Kidney beans	½ cup	4.5	Cabbage, raw	1 cup	2.2
Carrots, cooked	1 cup	4.4	Cucumbers	1 cup	2.2
Squash, summer	1 cup	4.4	Peaches	2 medium	2.0
White beans	½ cup	4.2	Cauliflower, cooked	1 cup	1.8
Lentils	½ cup	3.7	Tangerine	1 medium	1.8
Brussels sprouts	1 cup	3.6	Cherries	1 cup	1.7
Pear	1 medium	3.5	Onions, cooked	½ cup	1.6
String beans	1 cup	3.4	Pineapple	1 cup	1.6
Banana	1 medium	3.2	Walnuts	¼ cup	1.6
			Lima beans, dried	½ cup	1.4
			Tomato	1 medium	1.4

Sources: "Composition of Foods Commonly Used in Diets for Persons with Diabetes," *Diabetes Care,* September/October, 1978.

McCance and Widdowson's The Composition of Foods, by A. A. Paul and D. A. T. Southgate (New York: Elsevier/North-Holland Biomedical Press, 1978).

syrup, corn sweetener, natural sweetener, invert sugar, or honey—all terms used to describe various sugars. Sugar by any other name is just as sweet, just as devoid of vitamins and minerals, and thanks to such sweet deception, getting harder and harder to avoid. So read the labels carefully.

Calories: A Burning Issue

And if processed foods contain lots of sugar, it should come as no big surprise that they also are loaded with calories. People with arthritis have a particularly hard time with excess calories. Chances are, they're not moving around as much as they used to, or as much as they should. As a result, they don't burn up many calories in a day. Why, sitting quietly, crocheting, sewing by hand, or eating, for that matter, burn up less than half of 1 calorie each, if you perform the task for an hour. Dishwashing uses up only 1 calorie; painting furniture, 1½; walking slowly for an hour uses up only 2 mingy calories and vacuuming the rug only 2.7.

To avoid weight gain, you have to burn up all the calories you eat in a day. If you are unable to exercise strenuously, you probably won't be able to accomplish that goal. Therefore, you have to cut down on the number of calories you take in. For some people, such a reduction would mean giving up eating almost entirely, thus becoming deficient in important vitamins and minerals.

However, there are some dietary tricks you can try. Like an advertising campaign that wants to get "the most bang for the buck," you'll want to choose foods that offer the most nutrition for each calorie. Also choose foods that are filling but not fattening. There's no room at all in the diet for empty calories—as you find in sugar or alcohol. Moreover, think in terms of whole, natural, unprocessed foods, which contain every bit of nutrition they were meant to have.

Here are some rather dramatic examples of caloric equivalents:

   2 tablespoons of sugar = 5 cups of shredded cabbage
   1 tablespoon of mayonnaise = 40 spears of asparagus
   1 tablespoon of butter = 4 heads of lettuce

Table 5:   **ADDED SUGAR IN PROCESSED FOODS**

Food	Serving Size	Calories per Serving	Tea-spoons of Sugar per Serving	Percent of Calories
Wheaties	1 cup	110	0.7	11
Apple Jacks	1 cup	110	4.0	56
Sugar Smacks	¾ cup	110	4.0	56
Quaker 100% Natural Cereal	¼ cup	140	1.5	17
Blue cheese salad dressing	1 tablespoon	75	0.2	5
French salad dressing	1 tablespoon	65	0.7	18
Cranberry sauce	½ cup	203	11.7	90
Beef bologna	2 slices	150	0.3	4
Hot dogs	1	140	0.3	4
Yogurt, fruit	8 ounces	231	7.5	50
Beets, pickled	½ cup	57	2.1	57
Sweet peas, canned	½ cup	75	0.9	20

SOURCE: Adapted from *Nutrition Action*, August, 1979.

To help you make the switch to a more nutritious, less fattening diet, consider substituting the accompanying list of convenience equivalents. For each processed food, a substitute is listed that is nutritionally superior and less fattening, but just as convenient to prepare.

It's worth the effort to cut calories from the diet. Obesity is clearly related to diabetes, gallbladder disease, and high blood pressure. In association with other risk factors, it can contribute significantly to heart disease. With arthritis, you don't need any more health problems.

Table 6:   CONVENIENCE EQUIVALENTS

Instead of:	Try:
sweetened cereal	whole grain flakes with wheat germ
frozen waffles or pancakes with butter and syrup	whole wheat toast topped with applesauce
pizza	tuna packed in water
fatty lunch meat	blender shake of skim milk, fruit (or orange juice), and egg; if the blender pitcher is too heavy, just drop a straw right into it and enjoy
frozen, breaded fish or chicken	broiled filet of fish or breast of chicken
canned or frozen vegetables	fresh; if trimming or slicing is difficult, try fresh or steamed sprouts
canned or frozen fruit in syrup	yogurt with fresh fruit
pastry or cake	bran or corn muffin
cookies, crackers, candy	grapes, berries, or any fruit you can handle
coffee, tea, soda	fruit juice or spicy herb tea

9

THE HIDDEN HUNGER OF CELLS: NUTRITIONAL SUPPLEMENTS

Controversy surrounds the idea of using vitamins and minerals to ease the pain of arthritis. Many arthritics swear by some particular dietary regimen. Most doctors will tell you that vitamins probably won't do your illness a bit of good, but "if you feel better taking them, go ahead." The Arthritis Foundation, however, has vigorously opposed the use of vitamins and minerals as a form of arthritis therapy. The foundation's senior vice president of medical affairs, Frederic C. McDuffie, M.D., says in a foundation press release, "Most diet cures or super vitamin claims are outright quackery. All the individual gets for his trouble is false hopes and wasted money."

Dr. McDuffie's statement is not a one-time potshot at nutrition, but represents the foundation's historic stand on this issue. Year after year, this nationwide fund-raising group has repeated this belief, with modest variations, in its free and widely distributed pamphlet, *Arthritis: The Basic Facts*. Whether you read a pamphlet that's hot off the presses or years old, it will conclude, "The simple fact is, there is no scientific evidence that any food or vitamin deficiency has anything to do with causing arthritis and no evidence that any food or vitamin is effective in treating or 'curing' it."

Indeed, scientific evidence once was lacking. However, nutrition is a very young field of study. As recently as the

1940s, scientists were still discovering and naming new vitamins. Much of the early work in nutrition focused on finding deficiency diseases (like scurvy or pellagra) and setting recommended levels of vitamin consumption to prevent deficiencies. However, as this field of study matured, scientists began to delve into the more subtle and elusive roles of vitamins and minerals. How they are absorbed into the body and used, how they can interact with each other, their effect on the individual cells that make up our "whole"—all were studied.

As the investigation into nutrition continued, several intriguing facts emerged about the relationship between diet and arthritis. Studies have shown that people with arthritis are frequently deficient in some nutrient, even though they don't necessarily have the symptoms of any of the traditional deficiency diseases. Moreover, when their diets provided plenty of whatever the missing nutrient happened to be, people with arthritis began to improve. (More about specific vitamins and minerals later in this chapter.)

The Arthritis Foundation, however, has turned its back on these findings, instead repeating the notion that diet and arthritis have nothing to do with each other. It's ironic that the same group continues to support the use of expensive and sometimes dangerous drugs that treat only the symptoms of arthritis, but not the problem itself.

When asked what scientific evidence supports the contention that diet and arthritis have nothing to do with each other, one of the foundation's directors, Ann Fettner, said, "Hundreds of studies, none of which show a cause-and-effect relationship between diet and arthritis."

Of those hundreds, the foundation singled out *one* source—a study funded in part by the foundation itself. Called "Diet Therapy for Rheumatoid Arthritis" the foundation says this study is proof positive that there's no correlation between diet and arthritis.

Well, here's the study. Researchers at the University of Florida, Gainesville, put 30 people with rheumatoid arthritis (RA) on one of two diets for ten weeks. One of the diets, developed by Collin H. Dong, M.D., had been the subject of a book and was widely publicized in newspapers and magazines. It consists of almost no meat except for some fish and occasional fowl, no fruit, no herbs or spices, no dairy products, no alcoholic beverages, no additives, and no preservatives. The second diet was similar to Dr. Dong's, in that it also eliminated certain foods. Both diets provided the Recommended Dietary Allowances (RDA) of vitamins and minerals (levels which many doctors and nutritionists believe are too low for anyone, and may be particularly low for people with arthritis).

At the end of the ten-week test, nine patients had improved—five on the Dong diet, four on the second diet. Doctors who evaluated the results drew two conclusions. One, that the Dong diet, as followed for ten weeks by a small group of outpatients with long-standing progressive RA "was of no demonstrable benefit." Two, that "it is still possible that individualized dietary manipulations may be beneficial for selected patients with rheumatic disease."

And *this* is the study the Arthritis Foundation cites as proof positive there is no correlation between diet and nutrition.

The Way It Is

However, a quick scan of medical literature dealing with the topic of arthritis and nutrition quickly reveals the following new, startling, and very promising studies:

• At Wayne State University, in Detroit, Michigan, doctors have found that people with RA who followed a low-fat diet got better. Still on the diet, they have remained symptom-free for more than a year (more about this in chapter 10).

• Another study, this at the University of Texas, Austin, has found that one form of arthritis, carpal tunnel syndrome, is actually caused by a *vitamin deficiency*. The vitamin in this case is pyridoxine (B_6).

• A study at the University of Washington, Seattle, reported in the prestigious British journal, *Lancet,* shows that patients with RA had less joint swelling and stiffness when they took zinc.

• Another study on zinc, this at the University of Copenhagen, Denmark, and reported in the *British Journal of Dermatology,* shows that people with psoriatic arthritis improved significantly when their diet was supplemented with zinc. The study concludes, "Oral zinc sulphate seems to be invaluable in the treatment of psoriatic arthritis."

• In Israel, two doctors found that vitamin E provides "marked relief from pain in osteoarthritis."

• Yet other studies have reported that people with arthritis often have low levels of vitamin C.

Let's take a closer look at the link between arthritis and nutrition. While nobody can claim a sure cure for this dreadful disease, good nutrition certainly cannot hurt. And after all, vitamins and minerals are much, much safer than even aspirin, the most commonly used arthritis drug.

Exciting News about B_6

Important new research shows that one type of arthritis, carpal tunnel syndrome, is caused by a nutritional deficiency of vitamin B_6. Karl Folkers, Ph.D., director of the Institute for Biomedical Research at the University of Texas at Austin, recently announced this conclusion after six years of research.

Carpal tunnel syndrome usually affects the wrist. In fact, *carpus* is the medical word for your wrist. The bones and ligaments in your wrist form a tunnel through which pass the tendons and the nerves that make it possible for you to move your fingers and that control your sense of touch.

"When the disease strikes, an accumulation of fluid inside the carpal tunnel puts pressure on the nerve," explains Dr. Folkers. "This, in turn, leads to numbness and tingling in the tips of the fingers. Sometimes patients will tell me that at night their arms or hands 'fall asleep.' It's true that they may have, indeed, been sleeping on their arm, but I suspect that a more likely explanation is that they have carpal tunnel syndrome."

For years, patients with this disorder were routinely subjected to hand surgery to relieve compression on the nerve. But it's no secret that the surgery may only be partially successful and that any relief gained is likely to be lost in a few months.

Now, permanent relief of carpal tunnel syndrome is perhaps only a B_6 supplement away, thanks to the research efforts of Dr. Folkers and his associates. They were able to reach that conclusion by using a new and better blood test, which can detect and accurately measure deficiencies of vitamin B_6 on a patient-by-patient basis. Working in conjunction with John Ellis, M.D., of Mt. Pleasant, Texas, the doctors discovered that patients with carpal tunnel syndrome actually had an unrecognized, severe deficiency of vitamin B_6. What's more, B_6 supplements always corrected the deficiency and led to disappearance of the signs and symptoms.

Their next step was to repeat this research using the highly respected double-blind crossover technique. That means neither the patients nor the doctors conducting the experiments know which patients receive the actual vitamin and which receive a nontherapeutic, look-alike placebo pill, until the testing is completed.

Results? Patients responded well to the B_6 and not at all to the placebo. But when the patients on the placebo were given B_6, they, too, showed the same marked improvement.

"We've gotten as far as relating the disease to a B_6 deficiency and showing that the disease, if it hasn't progressed to the point of atrophy (wasting away), responds well to B_6," Dr. Folkers said. "And what I think is almost unbelievable (but it seems to be true) is that individuals who have had symptoms for years—a decade, even 15 years—show such remarkable reversal and improvement of their condition. I don't mean to say that the symptoms are 100 percent reversed, but they are improved so much that the patients do not need orthopedic surgery for their hands."

RDA IS "FAR TOO LOW"

"It doesn't even take huge doses of B_6, either," Dr. Folkers asserted. "However, I am convinced that the Recommended Dietary Allowance (RDA) of 2 milligrams is far too low. Our research shows that a very high percentage of the population in this country appears to have a deficiency of B_6. I believe that an effective RDA would be around 25 milligrams, or possibly even 35 milligrams. That means a supplement of B_6 will be needed to ensure health. In fact, the risk to health in not taking a B_6 supplement is far greater than the risk of taking it. Besides, it's virtually impossible to get that much B_6 in your daily diet," even if you eat foods rich in this nutrient, such as bananas, salmon, chicken, liver, and sunflower seeds.

Maybe you wonder whether you're deficient in vitamin B_6. There's actually a way you may be able to find out without even taking a laboratory test. Perhaps you've heard of a pesky health problem called the Chinese restaurant syndrome. It comes on about 20 minutes after eating a meal spiced heavily with monosodium glutamate (MSG). Headache, feverish flush, and a "detached or distant" feeling overcome those who are susceptible.

According to Dr. Folkers, it is people deficient in B_6 that develop the Chinese restaurant syndrome. He proved his theory by showing that supplemental B_6 could effectively prevent a recurrence of the MSG reaction, whereas a placebo had no effect.

Because of that study, Dr. Folkers began to wonder if those with carpal tunnel syndrome might also be sensitive to MSG, since they, too, have a B_6 deficiency. An opportunity became available in the case of a student who was known to be severely affected by carpal tunnel syndrome and extremely deficient in B_6.

Dr. Folkers was afraid the student might overreact to the 8.5 grams of MSG usually given in the test, so he cut the dosage to 4 grams, even though 4 grams rarely produced a response with other volunteers. Nevertheless, after 20 minutes, the predictable signs of Chinese restaurant syndrome appeared.

"The carpal tunnel syndrome reveals a vitamin B_6 deficiency over months and years," says Dr. Folkers, "but the Chinese restaurant syndrome reveals a deficiency over a period of 20 to 60 minutes. In principle, the underlying cause of both syndromes appears identical."

FOR HEBERDEN'S NODES

In addition to this deficiency disease, vitamin B_6 may also be helpful in treating Heberden's nodes, those bony lumps that form at finger joints in osteoarthritis. In fact, Jonathan V. Wright, M.D., of Kent, Washington, calls this particular ailment "pyridoxine-responsive arthritis." He tells the story of treating one patient with such a problem—a patient who was tired of taking painkillers but didn't want to live with pain.

The woman had arthritis in her fingers for several years, with X rays showing it in the slight to moderate range. "It was time to start doing something about her problem, and the answer was right in her hands," said Dr. Wright. "Almost everyone with this arthritis subtype improves with treatment centered around pyridoxine (B_6). As her hands were typical in appearance, I saw no reason why she shouldn't improve as others have."

The doctor recommended starting with 200 milligrams of pyridoxine, three times a day, backed up with a B-complex tablet including 50 milligrams of each of the B's, three times a day. After a month on this program the doctor reported that his patient had improved greatly. "The pain in her hands was more than 50 percent better. Her other aches and pains—in her shoulder, knee, and hip—were gone. And she was down to taking 6 aspirin daily, from 16." After several months of treatment, Dr. Wright's patient also was able to cut in half the amount of vitamin B_6 she was taking.

Niacinamide as Medicine

"Most doctors honestly believe that vitamins given in megadoses are a waste. They still think of vitamins in terms of the classical deficiency diseases, such as scurvy, beriberi, and pellagra. They are not thinking of lesser degrees of symptom-producing vitamin deficiencies that may also impair health. As an internist, I worked from the standpoint of always doing what I could for the health of my patients." These are the words of William Kaufman, M.D., Ph.D., a pioneer in the use of niacinamide as a treatment for arthritis.

"When I began practicing medicine in 1941, before the compulsory enrichment of cereal products in 1943, I realized that there was something going on that was a bit unusual. I found it striking that patient after patient came in with a group of symptoms and more subtle physical problems which were quite similar. They might have other symptoms besides. But in these certain symptoms, such as joint complaints, the lack of ability to concentrate, depression, irritability, excessive fatigue, bloating, and intestinal complaints, there was fingerprint similarity. Many patients were easily startled, so they jumped when the phone rang. A number had black and blue marks on their bodies where they had bumped into things since their balance sense was far off.

"I began tabulating symptoms that these men, women, and children had and very soon recognized that this strange syndrome was probably a form of pellagra, or niacin (which converts to its usable form, niacinamide) deficiency, that had not yet reached the degree of severity to cause the classic combination of skin rash, diarrhea, and dementia.

"I reasoned if this was a form of pellagra, then niacinamide—a B-complex vitamin which had then just been discovered as a preventive—might provide useful treatment. I prescribed it in very small doses at first, amounting to about 100 milligrams a day. Male and female patients would return a few days later and I didn't believe it! They looked different. They acted different. They told me that their symptoms had vanished, they felt a new zest for life. I decided to test it. I gave a few of these improved patients calcium instead of niacinamide. They were unaware of this change in their medication. At the end of ten days, they were right back to where they had been when they first saw me. When they resumed niacinamide treatment, they once more improved in the previous manner."

RESULTS ARE WHAT COUNT

Dr. Kaufman continued, "At first, the only test I had was the therapeutic test. Do the symptoms go away with the treatment? If you stop the treatment, do the symptoms come back? Of course, when calcium was substituted for niacinamide, the patient didn't know the treatment was stopped. Yet his symptoms returned. Then, when niacinamide therapy was resumed again, the symptoms disappeared. This was a good test.

"But even though I had good therapeutic results with this group of patients, I wasn't satisfied. I wanted to have a way of measuring improvements objectively. I needed some new standards of measurement. So I designed some simple instruments to measure joint mobility, and adapted other instruments for measuring muscle strength and working capacity. With these devices I could show, for example, how niacinamide enabled people to turn their heads further, as well as move their other joints through wider ranges of motion.

"The other instruments enabled me to measure people's strength and their working capacity. That told me whether they became tired more easily than normal. In addition, I used a biomicroscope to examine the tissue surfaces of the tongue, gums, lips, conjunctivae, and the cervix before and during treatment. To document what I saw, I took Kodachrome pictures with a special camera before and during treatment and in this way could check on the response of these tissues to treatment.

"Starting about 1943 with the compulsory enrichment of cereal products, fewer patients had the more severe symptoms. But measurements still showed many with joint dysfunction, decreased strength and muscle working capacity. Many of these benefited from treatment with niacinamide and other vitamins.

"I reported many of my findings to the medical profession by reading papers at the Second and Third International Congresses of Gerontology which were held in St. Louis and London respectively and before the Gerontological Society in Boston."

Despite Dr. Kaufman's presentations before medical societies, as well as publications describing his use of niacinamide, most doctors did not believe that vitamins as he used them could be of any help. However, numerous other doctors have agreed with his findings, including two surgeons whose careers were saved by Dr. Kaufman's treatment.

"Each surgeon thought he would have to give up his profession. Neither could manage the scissors or the scalpel proficiently. The reason was that their hands had become arthritic, stiff, and painful. Aspirin and other drugs failed to provide benefit.

"After three months of appropriate levels of niacinamide, the hands of both of these doctors improved so much that they were again able to function well as surgeons. One of them lived into his 80s and continued doing surgery until he was 75."

The daily doses of niacinamide Dr. Kaufman prescribed until the compulsory enrichment of bread in 1943 usually varied from 150 to 1,600 milligrams a day in divided doses. However, since 1944, the initial prescription usually was from 900 to 4,000 milligrams of niacinamide in divided doses a day. The selection of starting dosage regimen was based on the patient's initial Joint Range Index, the weighted average of the measured maximum ranges of joint motion of 20 specified joints. The dose was spread out throughout the day and no single dose ever exceeded 250 milligrams.

For niacinamide to be effective, the patient had to eat a diet adequate in protein and calories and not subject his joints to repetitive trauma, severe trauma, or overuse. Joints that are so severely damaged by the arthritic process that they represent end-stage joint disease have little or no capacity to recover joint mobility. Niacinamide is not a cure-all. However, most people treated with niacinamide have measurably improved joint mobility. Improvement is retained as long as the niacinamide regimen continues, the diet meets the required needs, and joints are not overused or injured.

Dr. Kaufman emphasizes the niacinamide treatment he has developed is *not* for self-treatment. The use of niacinamide in the manner prescribed by Dr. Kaufman should *always* be conducted under a doctor's supervision. The individualized niacinamide therapy for joint dysfunction as used by Dr. Kaufman's patients has been well tolerated and free from adverse side effects even when taken for decades.

Vitamin E for Pain Relief

Two Israeli doctors say vitamin E apparently gives "marked relief of pain" to some people with osteoarthritis.

In their experiment, 29 patients—4 men and 25 women—at Hasharon Hospital were assigned to either a group taking 600 International Units (I.U.) of vitamin E a day or a group taking an identical but inert pill. At the end of the experiment, fully 15 of the 29 "experienced marked relief of pain" while taking vitamin E, while only 1 of 29 patients had such a reaction to the placebo.

That's especially significant when you consider that these patients had been living with their woes for an average of over nine years.

Now, to what may we attribute these findings? It sure beats the doctors. I. Machtey, M.D., and L. Ouaknine, M.D., wrote in the *Journal of the American Geriatrics Society,* "The beneficial influence of tocopherol (the technical name for E) on joint symptoms in osteoarthritis cannot be explained at present." They take a stab at a possible explanation or two—tocopherol's anti-inflammatory potential, perhaps?—and wrap up with a modest proposal: "It would seem that further studies of this subject are warranted." (While we wait for the scientists to figure things out, you might want to try a private "study" on yourself.)

Scurvy: A Form of Arthritis

Everyone knows that scurvy will develop if we don't consume enough vitamin C. But hardly anyone realizes that scurvy is a form of arthritis. With this deficiency disease, blood oozes from the blood vessels and collects in the body's joints. The joints then become very painful and stiff. This joint problem is a major symptom and problem of scurvy. Of course, it can be prevented or cured with proper amounts of vitamin C.

Clearly, scurvy is different from other forms of arthritis, where the pain and swelling are the result of inflammation rather than bleeding. Even so, vitamin C may help these other types as well. For instance, researchers at Trinity College in Dublin, Ireland, have found that people with RA may need more vitamin C in their diets than healthy people. They reached this conclusion after comparing 42 people who had rheumatoid arthritis with 21 people who did not. Tests were given to measure the quantity of vitamin C in the blood. Among people with RA, 85 percent had levels well below normal. In fact, levels were *so low* they qualified for a diagnosis of *subclinical scurvy*. Researchers investigated the possibility that those with RA might be excreting more vitamin C than those in the healthy group. However, they soon found that was not the case. Researchers concluded their report on the study by saying, "It therefore appears that rheumatoid patients can absorb the vitamin at the same rate as normal (healthy) subjects. However, since intake and excretion of the vitamin did not differ between the groups it is probable that rheumatoid subjects utilize ascorbic acid at a faster rate."

In other words, an amount of vitamin C considered adequate for health may be totally *in*adequate for those with RA. How much is enough? This study did not attempt to find out. But since vitamin C plays an important role in maintaining the strength and functional capacity of every tissue in the body, it makes sense that it might help someone with the disease in which these very things are attacked.

Moreover, another study reveals that the effectiveness of aspirin, the mainstay of arthritis treatment, may be increased with vitamin C. Here's what happened. Researchers at the Simon Fraser University in Canada worked with human cells taken from both arthritic and healthy synovial fluid, as well as with some bone and muscle cells taken from laboratory animals. They cultured these cells with a combination of aspirin, vitamin C, and vitamin E.

The effect of aspirin alone on arthritic synovial cells was good, reducing the growth of these cells to an average of just 23 percent as compared to 100 percent growth of the cells not cultured with aspirin. But when vitamin C was added to the aspirin, the combination was *deadly* to the arthritis cells. They achieved zero growth. Further good news is that the aspirin/vitamin C mix did *not* affect the growth of cells that were not rheumatoid.

The Value of Zinc

"Many Americans may be consuming only marginally adequate levels of zinc," says a study on the zinc intake of elderly persons, reported in the *Journal of the American Dietetic Association*. The researchers who conducted the study measured the amount of zinc in the diet of a group of people with an average age of 69. They found that most of them were getting less than two-thirds of the RDA for zinc.

A similar study of people with an average age of 75 showed that even though their diet contained adequate levels of every *other* nutrient, they were getting less than two-thirds of the RDA for zinc.

These deficiencies are not limited to older folk. Other studies have been done on high school girls, who were revealed to be getting only one-third of the zinc they needed; and on children from middle- and low-income families, who were shown to be suffering from zinc malnutrition.

But why should *you* care about how much zinc you get? Because zinc may be a valuable treatment for arthritis.

One study in particular is extremely encouraging. It indicates that zinc deficiency may contribute to RA, and that treatment with zinc can reduce joint pain, swelling, and stiffness.

The study involved two groups; one was given zinc, the other a placebo. During the 12 weeks of the study, those taking zinc began to feel much better. Their joint swelling went down. They could walk faster. Their morning stiffness didn't last as long.

Peter A. Simkin, M.D., who conducted the study at the University of Washington, Seattle, theorized that low zinc levels cause RA to be more active. "Zinc supplementation," he concluded, "would reverse this process, inhibit the inflammatory response, and thereby ameliorate the effects of the disease."

Dr. Simkin suggested more research on zinc. And five years later, another report on its beneficial effects appeared in the medical press. The good news, according to researchers at the University of Copenhagen, Denmark, is that

112

zinc can make most of the symptoms of psoriatic arthritis disappear. People who took zinc found a "significant reduction" of morning stiffness as well as generally feeling better all over. Moreover, they were able to cut down on the amount of painkilling medication taken. Most of the joints involved in the disease were less swollen and more flexible. Unfortunately, the zinc didn't clear up the psoriasis—just the joint inflammation. But for many that would be good enough!

A Powder to Halt Bone Loss

One of the long-term effects of RA is bone loss. At times, the loss is so severe it actually can result in broken bones. It seems the bones become so thin and weak they simply fracture. Doctors have known about this problem for a very long time, but little has been done to prevent it. In fact, the frequently prescribed drugs such as cortisone and other steroids actually speed bone loss and promote breaks!

In England, doctors recently tried giving patients with RA a daily supplement of bone powder to see if it would help. Some 72 people—all over 50 and taking steroid drugs—were divided into two groups. One group took 6 grams of bone powder each day and continued taking their prescribed medication. The bone powder provided substantial amounts of calcium as well as other minerals and trace elements. The second group just took the steroids.

After 12 months, the people were measured for height loss (a result of broken vertebrae) and bone density. The group that did not take the bone powder lost much more height and bone density than the people who were lucky enough to be chosen for the other group. A lot of medical men would predict health problems after taking so much calcium every day for a whole year, particularly a condition called hypercalciuria. But nobody taking the special powder developed this "overdose-of-calcium" disease.

While the underlying RA seemed about the same for both sets of people, you wouldn't guess that from talking to them. Those who didn't take calcium complained *three times as much* about back pain as those who did.

In another British study, investigators determined that a

vitamin D deficiency was causing both the bone loss and fractures common to people with RA. These investigators discovered that, partly due to finances, the folks under study had not been eating foods high in vitamin D, such as margarine, sardines, and milk. The resulting vitamin D deficiency was, they said, responsible for these bone problems. They suggested that a supplement of 300 I.U. of vitamin D would prevent the deficiency, and presumably, the broken bones, as well.

Nourishing the Cells

What are we to make of all these findings? The medical establishment says all these studies to date don't amount to a hill of beans. Yet many people have been helped by these vitamins and minerals. How *do* you explain it? Biochemist E. C. Barton-Wright, D.Sc., a physician at the Rheumatic Clinic at St. Alfege's Hospital, London, says, "All vitamins are equally important in the complex chain of chemical reactions that take place in our bodies. It is the *quantitative* aspect that is all important. In other words, are our bodies taking in sufficient amounts of these substances daily?" He concludes that the amounts required to maintain health and well-being vary from individual to individual . . . "a fact that has been entirely ignored by the statisticians and medical profession."

For arthritis in particular, it may be that certain crucial cells necessary for the proper functioning of the joints have specific needs that are not being met in our everyday diets. Take joint cartilage, for example. It is made of a unique tissue that must be smooth and slippery so the joints can flex, and yet be strong enough to not only bear the weight of our bodies but stand up under the pressure of our daily activities. This cartilage is made up mainly of collagen, a fiberlike protein substance. The second major component of cartilage is something called "ground substance." Without getting into a complicated discussion of biochemistry to explain how these two elements of cartilage use the various nutrients in our bodies, let's just note that healthy collagen requires sufficient vitamin C and copper. Ground substance, the element that is believed to provide firmness and moisture to cartilage, requires vitamin C to interact with collagen. Other nutrients are required by the glands that influence the breakdown and replacement of collagen and other connective tissue.

The optimum diet would feed these tissues adequately. And, as Dr. Barton-Wright points out, each of us has special, individual requirements for each vitamin and mineral. Those who want to pursue nutrition as a therapy for arthritis should consult Appendix 1 for a list of physicians and other health professionals who have expressed an interest in providing this (or another holistic alternative) to people with arthritis. Or you could try some of these therapies on your own. In either case, you may find that nutrients are an important part of arthritis relief.

10

ARTHRITIS DIETS: FACT OR FICTION?

Some of the most fascinating reading can be found in the "Letters to the Editor" columns of our country's prestigious medical journals. Here doctors offer the medical equivalent of household hints, swap "trade secrets," and hold forth on the state of their art.

For example, a recent issue of the *New England Journal of Medicine* published a letter from a doctor practicing in a rural community in Maine. He said he knew of a farmer who had heart problems. The man was plagued by an irregular, runaway beat. One day the farmer showed up at the doctor's office and proclaimed that he'd found a cure for his problem. Seems he accidentally stumbled into the electrified wire fence he uses to contain his dairy herd. When his chest hit the wire he got a mild shock and—lo and behold!—his heart began beating steadily. After that experience, every time he felt a recurrence of that distressing syncopated beat, he'd head out to the pasture and give himself a little jolt. The farmer was so pleased with the effectiveness of the treatment that he was having an electrified wire strung across his basement so he wouldn't have to walk so far for help.

The doctor mused, "As remarkable as his story is, what made the greatest impression was that if I hadn't known that an electric shock passed across the chest could effectively resolve cardiac arrhythmias (irregular beat), I most probably would have dismissed his tale as so much colorful folklore. In that context, I have to wonder what other potentially useful therapeutic modalities have been similarly dismissed by me and my learned colleagues."

Perhaps such is the case with several diets that work to relieve arthritis pain, swelling, and stiffness. Most doctors honestly and firmly believe that what you eat has absolutely no effect on your arthritis. Yet people on these diets often find relief. Fortunately, a small number of doctors have come forward to explain how certain specific diets really may help almost everyone with arthritis. These range from a low-fat diet that has cleared up the symptoms of active rheumatoid arthritis (RA), to individually designed allergy diets for people suffering from *all* forms of arthritis, to a diet developed by a horticulturist who found that certain poisons which naturally exist in some vegetables may cause arthritis agony.

The Amazing Low-Fat Diet

One of the most promising of these diets has been devised by two doctors at Wayne State University in Detroit, Michigan. They backed into a remarkable discovery while they were working with obese patients on a low-fat diet. Two of the group had active RA. Amazingly, after just five days on the special diet, their arthritis symptoms disappeared and have not returned as long as they have stayed on it.

"Now, I don't believe this diet affects the basic, underlying rheumatoid disease," says Lawrence Power, M.D., co-developer of the diet. "However, the body needs fat to produce the intermediary products like prostaglandins that fuel inflammation. Take away the fuel and you take away the inflammation."

Dr. Power and his colleague, Charles P. Lucas, M.D., are quite enthusiastic about the benefits of this diet. "It all began with one patient who had long-standing arthritis. Her condition—in her hands, mostly—cleared up on the diet. After a while, she went back to regular food and discovered the inflammation had returned. At first we suspected that meat was the culprit. But it wasn't. The problem, we soon learned, was fat in any form."

Soon, the doctors discovered a second patient at the clinic also had RA. That condition, too, cleared quickly. The doctors then "borrowed" several RA patients from a colleague who is also a rheumatologist. With this small group of 6, they again duplicated their remarkable results. At this writing, Drs. Power and Lucas are working with 30 arthritis patients.

"Nearly all are symptom-free as long as they remain on the diet. One patient couldn't resist blue cheese dressing on her salad, and suffered with RA pain for three days afterward. Now, not absolutely everyone on this diet will improve, but nine out of ten will," Dr. Power explains.

How has the medical community received the good news? "They laughed and called us food faddists," Dr. Power says. The new study is under the direction of a rheumatologist, in an effort to legitimize the results so they will be taken seriously. Other tests also are under way, including one at the University of California.

THE PRITIKIN PROMISE

In the meantime, Nathan Pritikin has watched the results of his own low-fat diet on visitors at his Longevity Center in Santa Monica, California. The fact that Drs. Power and Lucas could "cure" arthritis with a diet almost identical to his own surprised Pritikin as much as if someone just told him that aspirin cures headaches.

"I've known about *that* for ten years," he said. And he has more than one fabulous tale to tell about arthritis and the low-fat diet. Surely, the most dramatic is the story of Eula Weaver.

"She came to the Center when she was 81 years old. She had severe rheumatoid arthritis which had terribly distorted her fingers. She also had angina, hypertension, and a host of other health problems. The arthritis in her right knee was so bad she couldn't walk up even one step. After one year on the low-fat diet, she was off all medication, her arthritis was disappearing, and her joint function had returned.

"When she was 85½ years old, she entered the Senior Olympics and won two gold medals; one for winning the one-mile race, and the other for winning the half-miler. She last raced when she was 90½ years old. In that ten-year period her arthritis completely disappeared," tells Pritikin.

Eula's case history is not isolated. Pritikin also recounts the story of a woman with excruciating pain in her fingers and another who gave up hope after 35 years of arthritis and drugs. Both are well today.

Unlike Dr. Power, Pritikin believes that the diet does strike at the disease itself and not just the inflammation. "The disease is not a mystery. Fat and salt are the primary cause, with fat the major factor. On a low-fat diet, the body has substantially better circulation. Fat coats the red blood cells so they can't get through the small blood vessels. This limited circulation lowers oxygen levels and indirectly destroys certain cells of the immune system, whose powerful enzymes then leak into the joint. The result is rheumatoid arthritis. Salt, meanwhile, causes the tissues to become flooded with water which also lessens circulation," Pritikin explains.

VERY FAST ACTING

If you would like to try the diet, all you've got to lose are your aches and pains and maybe some weight. Pritikin says it works on 90 percent of the people who have arthritis in their hands, fingers, and wrists, and on 50 percent of the people who have arthritis in their knees and hips. "Maybe we get them too late, after serious joint damage has already occurred," he muses. You'll know fairly soon if the diet is working for you. Most people begin to improve in one or two weeks and feel better in two to six weeks. (See Table 7.)

"It's not a matter of being overweight, but of eating too much fat," warns Pritikin. "Eula Weaver never weighed more than 110 pounds in her life."

Dr. Power agrees. "We love food that is moist, rich, and buttery," he says. "But we were never meant to eat fat the way we do—we were meant to eat it as it is found naturally in whole foods. Look at it this way: you'd have to eat an awful lot of corn to get one tablespoon of corn oil. It's important to adjust your thoughts about food so that when you're hungry you want an apple instead of a doughnut."

Thus, if you follow Dr. Power's line of reasoning, you'd stop eating cheese, butter, whole milk, red meat, pork, anything fried, most nuts and seeds, cakes, pastries, and so forth. Instead, you would load up on cereals and grains, skim milk, fruits, vegetables, and fish. If the cauşe of your arthritis pain is fat, you'll feel the intensity of your symptoms lessen in time. If the diet does not help your arthritis pain, at least it will have nourished you well, aided your digestion, unclogged your arteries, and slimmed your body. Surely there could be no harm in trying it.

Allergy and Arthritis

"A *minimum* of 80 percent of all people with rheumatoid arthritis have an allergic condition in their affected joints and surrounding structures that are involved in this disease," says Marshall Mandell, M.D., a Norwalk, Connecticut, allergist who practices clinical ecology. "Allergic reactions aggravate and perpetuate the swelling, redness, pain, and limitation of motion. I am convinced that allergic reactions are the underlying cause of many cases of this form of arthritis. Allergy also plays an important role in childhood arthritis and osteoarthritis." Along with colleague Anthony Conte, M.D., of Beaver, Pennsylvania, Dr. Mandell completed a study of 40 people with arthritis that revealed their arthritis symptoms, along with other important chronic ailments, were caused by reactions to frequently eaten foods or exposure to something in the environment they are allergic to.

"We investigated the relationship between arthritis and allergy in 40 volunteers with arthritis by means of a double-blind study, where neither the patients nor the doctors knew which substances were being tested on whom. We tested our volunteers for allergies with specially prepared solutions of food, house dust, molds, tobacco smoke, and petrochemicals. Eighty-six percent had arthritis symptoms—their usual chronic joint and muscle complaints—provoked by these allergens (substances that cause allergic reactions). The method of testing we employed was one that actually reproduced the volunteers' familiar symptoms. Most had no idea that allergies might be a very important factor in their illness," Dr. Mandell explained.

"The body's response to an allergen is complex and can involve arthritis, nervous system disorders, respiratory ail-

Table 7: **THE PRITIKIN PLAN: FOODS TO USE AND AVOID**

Category	Foods to Use	Quantity Permitted	Foods to Avoid
Fats and oils	None	None	All fats and oils, including butter, margarine, shortening, lard, meat fat, and lecithin (as in vegetable spray)
Sugars	None	None	All extracted sugars, including syrups, molasses, fructose, dextrose, sucrose, and honey
Poultry, fish, shellfish, and meat		Limit acceptable poultry, fish, and meat to a total of 1½ lbs./ week or 3½ oz./ day	All smoked, charbroiled, or barbecued foods
	Chicken, turkey, and Cornish game birds (white meat preferred; remove skin before cooking)		Fatty poultry: duck and goose
	Lean fish and shellfish	Lobster: 3½ oz./day (replaces entire daily allotment of poultry, fish, or meat)	Fatty fish: sardines, fish canned in oil, and mackerel

Category	Foods to Use	Quantity Permitted	Foods to Avoid
		Shrimp, oysters, crab, clams, or scallops: 1¼ oz./day (replaces entire daily allotment of poultry, fish, or meat)	
	Lean meat		Fatty meat: marbled steaks, fatty hamburger and other fatty ground meat, bacon, spareribs, sausage, hot dogs, lunch meat, etc.
			Organ meat: liver, kidney, heart, and sweetbread
Eggs	Egg whites	7/week maximum (raw: 2/ week maximum)	Egg yolks and fish eggs (caviar and shad roe)
Dairy foods	Nonfat milk (skim or buttermilk, up to 1% fat by weight) or nonfat yogurt	8 oz./day	Cream, half-and-half, whole milk, and low-fat milk, or products containing or made from them, such as sour cream or low-fat yogurt

Category	Foods to Use	Quantity Permitted	Foods to Avoid
	Nonfat (skim) powdered milk	5 level tsp./day (replaces entire allotment of fluid skim milk or equivalents)	Nondairy substitutes (creamers and whipped toppings)
	Evaporated skim milk	4 oz./day (occasional use only); replaces entire allotment of fluid skim milk or equivalents	
	100% skim milk cheeses (uncreamed cottage cheese, such as hoop cheese or dry-curd cottage cheese, or cheeses up to 1% fat by weight)	2 oz./day	Cheeses containing over 1% fat by weight
	Sapsago (green) cheese	1–2 oz./week maximum	
Beans and peas	All beans and peas (except soybeans)	Limit to 1–1½ lbs./week (cooked) maximum; in addition, may substitute 8- oz.serving	Soybeans, unless used as a substitute for poultry, fish, shellfish, or meat allotment (1 oz. soybeans = 1 oz. flesh)

Category	Foods to Use	Quantity Permitted	Foods to Avoid
		for each 3½-oz. serving of acceptable poultry, fish, shellfish, or meat	
		Limit to 2-oz. serving twice/ week substituted for day's cheese allotment or equivalent	
Nuts and seeds	Chestnuts	Not limited	All nuts (except for chestnuts)
			All seeds (except in small quantities for seasoning as with spices)
Vegetables	All vegetables except avocados and olives	Limit vegetables high in oxalic acid, such as spinach, beet leaves, rhubarb and Swiss chard	Avocados and olives
Desserts and snacks	Desserts and snack items without fats, oils, sugars, or egg yolks	Plain gelatin (unflavored): 1 oz./week maximum	Desserts and snack items containing fats, oils, sugars, or egg yolks, such as most bakery

Category	Foods to Use	Quantity Permitted	Foods to Avoid
			goods, package gelatin desserts and puddings, candy, chocolate, and gum
Condiments, salad dressings, sauces, gravies, and spreads	Wines for cooking Natural flavoring extracts Products without fats, oils, sugars, or egg yolks	Dry white wine preferable; moderate use	Products containing fats, oils, sugars, or egg yolks, such as mayonnaise, prepared sandwich spreads, prepared gravies and sauces, and most seasoning mixes, salad dressings, catsups, pickle relish, and chutney
Salt	Salt	Limit salt intake to 3–4 g./day by eliminating table salt and restricting use of high salt or sodium foods such as soy sauce, pickles, most condiments, prepared sauces, dressings, canned vegetables,	Salt from all sources in excess of permitted amount

Category	Foods to Use	Quantity Permitted	Foods to Avoid
		and MSG (monosodium glutamate)	
Grains	All whole or lightly milled grains: rice, barley, buckwheat, millet, etc.	Unlimited	Extracted wheat germ
	Breads, cereals, crackers, pasta, tortillas, baked goods, and other grain products without added fats, oils, sugars, or egg yolks	Limit refined grains and grain products (i.e., with bran and germ removed), such as white flour, white rice, white pasta, etc.	Grain products made with added fats, oils, sugars, or egg yolks Bleached white flour or soy flour
Fruit	All fresh fruit	5 servings/day maximum	
	Unsweetened cooked, canned, pureed, or frozen fruit	24 oz./week maximum	Cooked, canned, pureed, or frozen fruit with added sugars Jams, jellies, fruit butters, and fruit syrups with added sugars
	Dried fruit	1 oz./day maximum	

Category	Foods to Use	Quantity Permitted	Foods to Avoid
	Unsweetened fruit juices	4 oz./day maximum (28 oz./week)	Fruit juices with added sugars
	Frozen concentrates, undiluted	1 oz./day maximum (7 oz./week)	
Beverages	Mineral water and carbonated water	Limit variation with added sodium	Alcoholic beverages
	Nonfat (skim) milk or nonfat buttermilk	See restrictions under *Dairy foods*	Beverages with caffeine: coffee, tea, cola drinks, etc.
	Unsweetened fruit juices	See restrictions under *Fruit*	Beverages with added sweeteners such as soft drinks
	Vegetable juices	Carrot juice: 2 glasses/week maximum	Diet and other soft drinks with artificial sweetener
	Linden or Red Bush tea		

SOURCE: *The Pritikin Program for Diet and Exercise,* by Nathan Pritikin (New York: Grosset and Dunlap, 1979).

ments, gastrointestinal and urinary tract disorders, and even eye problems. My clinical experience indicates that at least 70 percent of the general population—about 150 million people in this country alone—suffer from some form of internal allergy that is unsuspected, unrecognized, undiagnosed, and, therefore, incorrectly treated. Each human being has a biologic uniqueness which is going to determine which substances will or will not cause health problems in a particular person. Much depends on the duration or amount of exposure to the allergen, exposure to indoor and outdoor air pollutants, chemical additives, a person's nutritional state, and so on. Some people will react to only one or two substances, others will respond to more than a dozen, and some individuals may be allergic to almost every food they eat."

According to Dr. Mandell, you should suspect your arthritis is allergy related if you have a strong family history of allergy, a personal history of allergy, or if your arthritis improves during a fast or illness, when you lose your appetite. You also should suspect allergy as the culprit if your arthritis gets worse on a certain day of the week, during a particular season, at a particular location, during some activity, after certain meals, after taking an alcoholic beverage, or after an obvious chemical exposure.

If you think your arthritis is allergy related, keep a careful record of your personal observations, noting when your arthritis got worse and what food or other substances you have been exposed to that may have provoked the attack. These observations often provide valuable clues to determining what your particular offending substances may be.

SUGGESTIONS FOR FOLLOWING THE PRITIKIN DIET

1. Eat 2 or more kinds of whole grain daily (wheat, oats, brown rice, barley, buckwheat, etc.) in the form of cereals, side dishes, pasta, bread, etc.

2. Eat 2 or more servings of raw vegetable salad and two or more servings of raw, or cooked, green or yellow vegetables daily. Potatoes may be eaten every day.

3. Eat 1 piece of citrus fruit and up to 3 or 4 fresh fruit servings daily.

4. Do not use sugar or honey of any kind. When sweeteners are necessary, use pureed fresh fruit or fruit juices.

5. Eat beans or peas 1 to 3 times weekly, as you wish.

6. Limit protein intake from animal* sources as follows:

> Up to 24 ounces per week of low-fat, low-cholesterol meat, fish, shellfish, or fowl.

> Up to 8 ounces (1 glass) skim milk and 2 ounces of uncreamed cottage cheese per day or equivalent in skim milk products.

7. If you have constipation problems, add some unprocessed wheat bran flakes (starting with 1 tablespoon daily) to your cereal, soup, or other foods.

8. Eat 3 full meals daily. Don't go hungry between meals; snacks are encouraged. For snacks, eat fruit (not exceeding daily fruit allotment), vegetables, and raw salad, or whole grain bread or crackers that are free of oil, fat, added wheat germ, or sweeteners.

9. Flavor with herbs and spices, instead of salt. Keep salt intake minimal.

10. If you need to lose weight, increase vegetables and decrease grains. If you need to gain weight, decrease vegetables and increase grains.

*Vegetarians eating no animal protein at all may require a supplement of vitamin B_{12} once every several weeks.

Armed with this information, you can set about eliminating these problem substances from your life. Unfortunately, some of the foods most likely to cause a problem are old favorites that will be missed. "But you don't have to avoid these foods forever," says Dr. Mandell. After your arthritis is under control, you will be able to eat many of them again without any problems, perhaps once every five to seven days.

After staying on your own individualized allergy-arthritis diet with great success, you may suddenly have a flare-up.

Why? Dr. Mandell suggests that perhaps the diet relied too heavily on a certain food, creating a new allergic sensitivity because of an overexposure to a troublemaker. Should this happen, do not feel the entire effort has been a failure. Instead, calmly determine which foods may be causing your problem, and eliminate them.

Dr. Mandell is not alone in his conviction that there is a connection between allergy and arthritis. In England, 20 out of 22 patients with RA who followed allergen-free diets found improvement in less than three weeks. Of the group, 14 were sensitive to grain, 8 to nuts and seeds, 7 to cheese, 5 to eggs, 4 each to milk and beef, and 1 each to chicken, fish, potato, onion, and liver.

NEW TEST, NEW CONTROVERSY

And in California, James Braly, M.D., head of Optimum Health Labs in Encino, has developed allergen-free diets that have successfully helped several famous athletes and relieved actor James Coburn of his severe arthritis pain. Dr. Braly uses a new and very controversial procedure to uncover individual allergies. Called the "cytotoxic food allergy test," a blood sample is centrifuged to remove the plasma and white cells. Next, tiny groups of these cells are mingled with individual food concentrates. In theory, if the person is allergic to a certain food, his white blood cells should change shape or even rupture after several hours' contact with that food sample concentrate.

Like Dr. Mandell, Dr. Braly says that each individual's reaction is unique, and thus, so is his allergy diet. "Arthritis, like other degenerative diseases, is a multifactorial disease," he says. He also believes the diet, along with supplements and exercise, will cure a host of ills. In an interview with *Muscle & Fitness* magazine, he said, "Within a few weeks of eliminating the allergenic foods from your diet, you'll notice some drastic changes in your physical and psychological well-being. One immediate result is a marked weight loss. Some patients lose up to 10 to 15 pounds in two or three weeks. This is primarily water that's flushed from the system once the allergy-induced inflammations have abated.

"You'll notice that your irritability will gradually diminish, and all of the other allergy-related symptoms that you've noticed will also start to disappear. It may take several weeks, but even your arthritis problems will become a thing of the past."

Dr. Braly's multifactorial approach suggests the elimination of allergic foods; rotation of nonallergic foods; supplementation with vitamins, minerals, and trace minerals; and eating unprocessed, unrefined (or minimally refined), and chemically uncontaminated foods. "This may be *primary* in treatment of arthritis and other patients with degenerative disease, that is, assuring that *what* they eat and *how* they eat results in proper and complete digestion of foods. Evidence indicates that *many* people partially digest food and *frequently* absorb these partially digested foods into the bloodstream. Once in the bloodstream, these foods are treated *not* as nutrients but instead as allergens, toxins, or addictants.

"I strongly recommend that the person with arthritis stop alcohol, stop caffeine, stop tobacco, stop refined sugars and excess fats, stop food allergens, and learn to deal more effectively with mental stress. Moreover, I find that exercise is extremely important in treating arthritis."

The No-Nightshade Approach

The family of plants called nightshades (Solonaceae) has been linked with arthritis, rheumatism pain, and disfigurement by Norman F. Childers, Ph.D., a retired professor of horticulture. This botanical family includes two very poisonous members—the deadly and the black nightshades—which are used in drugs such as belladonna, atropine, and scopolamine. They're strong enough to kill you if you eat enough of them. If these were the only plants in the family it surely would be no trouble to avoid them. But there's a catch. The other members in the family are the white potato, tomato, eggplant, tobacco, and all pepper except black (a different family).

Dr. Childers says it's not an allergy problem that results from eating these foods but a toxic problem—a kind of slow poisoning. However, he claims that the plants don't bother everyone, but only about 5 to 10 percent of the population who are sensitive to chemicals such as solanine they all contain. Dr. Childers claims these toxins cause arthritis inflammation and pain.

He discovered the relationship between nightshades and joint pain on his own, after he stopped eating tomatoes for a time and noticed an improvement in his stiff neck. Although he is not a medical doctor, he plunged into medical research by launching a nationwide survey involving thousands of volunteers. Eventually, he published a book called *A Diet to Stop Arthritis* (Somerset Press, 1977).

The results of his survey are mixed but encouraging. Those who found improvement, some 72 percent, are very enthusiastic about the diet. For example, Arthur H. Thompson, Ph.D., of College Park, Maryland, says that even after 20 years of deterioration his condition improved remarkably. "I eliminated the nightshades from my diet, but I did so without conviction, with some desperation, perhaps, and with utterly nothing to lose. One by one, painful daily realities disappeared. For a time I could not believe what was happening to me—and did not. It simply couldn't be that easy.

"But it was. Incredibly, I was soon back to normal, painless activity I thought was gone forever for me. I could get out of bed or a chair normally. I could bend over and tie my shoelaces again. In just three months, the pain and restricted movement from 20 years of arthritis was gone! And it happened without a single aspirin. I simply had eliminated the nightshades from my diet. Even today I find it all quite amazing."

Dr. Childers says the diet is not as easy to follow as it looks because traces of these forbidden fruits are found in many processed foods. He believes the reason that many volunteers on the diet did not improve may be that they were still eating the nightshades without being aware of it, or using tobacco. For example, some inexpensive yogurts are thickened with potato starch and some packaged foods are colored with paprika.

Moreover, the diet must be followed *at least* three months—and often six to nine months—before results are seen. With his permission, we include a table that lists the most likely hiding places for these problem foods.

Table 8: **FOODS CONTAINING NIGHTSHADES**
(Always check ingredient labels.)

Potato In

Baby foods
(check label)

Biscuits (check
label)

Breads (check
label)

Chowder, clam

Consomme
(check label)

Doughnuts
(check label)

Fish cakes,
precooked
and/or frozen

Hash, meatballs,
meat loaf,
stews

Meat pies
(frozen): beef,
chicken, turkey

Sauce, taco

Soups (check
label)

Vegetables,
mixed (check
label)

Yogurt (check
label)

Tomato In

Baby foods (check
label)

Beans, baked,
canned

Beef stews, soups,
pies

Cabbage, stuffed,
frozen

Chicken, breading
mix

Chips, corn, tortilla

Chow mein, canned

Delicatessen foods
(many)

Dinners, frozen
(check label)

Fillets, herring
(check label)

Hamburger Helper

Italian foods: frozen,
dry, canned

Meat loaf

Rice, Spanish,
canned

Salad dressings

Salisbury steaks,
frozen

Sauces: barbecue,
cocktail,
spaghetti, steak,
taco

Soups (check label)

Vegetable juice,
mixed, canned

Peppers (Red or Green) In

Artichoke hearts, canned

Baby foods (check label)

Bologna

Bread crumbs (check label)

Crabs, deviled, frozen

Cauliflower, pickled, spiced

Chicken: canned or frozen,
hot take-out, chow mein,
breading mix

Chips, corn, tortilla

Crackers, seasoned

Delicatessen foods (sprinkled with paprika)

Dinners, frozen (check label)

Dips (check label)

Egg noodles, Chinese

Fillets, herring (check label)

Fish cakes, precooked and/ or frozen

Gravy (check label)

Ham glaze

Hot dogs

Italian foods: frozen, dry, canned

Kasha mix (check label)

Mayonnaise (check label)

Meat loaf, smoked lunch meat, tenderizers

Meat pies (frozen): beef, chicken, turkey

Olives, stuffed

Onion rings, frozen

Rarebit, Welsh

Relishes

Rice: Chinese, fried, seasoned, Spanish with sweet pepper bits

Salad dressings (check label)

Salts, some seasoned

Sardines in seasoned sauce

Sauces: barbecue, Sloppy Joe, Tabasco, taco (check label)

Sausage

Seasoning mixes

Shrimp: breaded, croquettes, scampi

Spices (check label)

Spreads: cracker, sandwich

Veal patties, frozen

Vegetables: frozen "international" mixes, frozen with sauce, Chinese, juices

---

NOTE: Other foods eaten in excess may cause problems. These include asparagus, beets, rhubarb, spinach, and particularly milk and products with vitamin D added, along with other items on the grocery shelves that also contain vitamin D, such as oleomargarine and breakfast cereals. Rather than relying upon only a few foods, it is better to eat and drink a wide variety from day to day.

Through the Closed Door

As you can see, these diets are quite different from each other. The endocrinologists treating people for obesity quite logically were drawn to a low-fat diet. The allergist, of course, developed individualized diets based on his own special interest. Needless to say, the horticulturist found the basis of his arthritis problem in his garden.

Thus, the information provided can be confusing. There has been little research on diet and arthritis, and the connection between the two has been pooh-poohed by the medical community at large; as a result, there is no broad overview to guide individual researchers.

If you want to try a diet to help relieve your arthritis, where do you begin? You begin by making some careful choices. If, for example, you do have some allergies, you might try Dr. Mandell's approach. If you eat fatty foods, then Dr. Power's and Nathan Pritikin's diets may be the place for you to start. And, if you can get through the day without potatoes, tomatoes, and such, try the no-nightshades approach.

These diets can do you no harm. They are certainly a much less expensive treatment than drugs. However, you will have to invest some time and patience. But the payback can be enormous!

11

WONDERFUL WATER

Water is the major component of our bodies, with each of our hundred trillion cells filled and bathed with it. It is the basis of our blood and our tears, and essential for each breath we take. Humanity has long recognized the somewhat mystical qualities of water, knowing that it does more than simply slake thirst. To Archimedes, Nero, and even the Mayas who built Chichén-Itzá, water was a common cure. The Emperor Hirohito and the Apache Chief Cochise—on opposite sides of the planet—both soothed their minds and muscles in a bath. Water, it seems, is the oldest and most universal of all healers.

Here at the end of the twentieth century, doctors and other health professionals still recommend water therapy. Why? Because it's economical, relaxing, and has no hidden side effects to sneak up on you later. And, of course, it works.

The ancient art of hydrotherapy uses water in all its forms—liquid, vapor, and solid. The right water treatment can relieve symptoms for any kind of arthritis, and is an absolute must for those with rheumatoid arthritis (RA). Moreover, aside from its pain-relieving function, hydrotherapy also can prevent (and sometimes even correct) deformities and improve joint function. However, this treatment doesn't work like a "miracle" drug. You don't just take two baths and feel better in the morning. Hydrotherapy requires some time and a committed effort on your part. But you should find the experience so pleasant and the results so rewarding that you'll actually look forward to each treatment.

If you were in a hospital, you would be placed in the care of a physical therapist. He or she might require you to spend some time in a Hubbard tank—a huge affair, shaped like a figure eight, with pulleys, straps, and levers that lower you into and out of the water. However, here we'll try to provide techniques for the same sort of therapy without all the scary-looking equipment. To work at home, you'll need a bathtub, two deep basins or bowls, an ice bag or an ordinary baggie, and—if possible—access to a swimming pool or a hot tub. (Yep, a hot tub!)

Water does amazing things for arthritis. If it's hot, it increases the blood flow in the joints and relieves muscle pain. Cold water increases muscle tone. In addition to the treatment of symptoms, you'll start to feel better in general.

For most people, the easiest place to begin hydrotherapy is in their own bathtub. Using a thermometer (one made for a tropical fish tank is okay), check to make sure the water temperature is between 100° and 102°F. By no means get into a tub of water hotter than 104°F. Your body won't be able to throw off enough of its own heat and you can suffer from hyperthermia—a kind of underwater heat prostration.

You don't need any special water for hydrotherapy. It would be nice to fill your tub each day with some marvelous elixir from a mineral spring, like those wonderful old European spas use. But most of us can't. Instead, just use whatever comes out of the tap.

If you're not sure you can get in and out of the tub safely, here's a simple technique that will help. Usually, most people just step into the tub facing the faucets and sit down. Instead, get into the tub facing the opposite end. Next, get down on your hands and knees. Slowly slide around into a sitting position, pressing one foot against the side of the tub to steady you and act as a pivot. To get out of the tub, first drain the water, then reverse the procedure.

Additionally, you should have no-slip treads installed on the bottom of the tub. And, if you require additional support, you can buy hand rails that affix to its sides. These can be found at medical supply stores or even at some well-equipped pharmacies.

Once in the bath, plan on staying there for 20 to 30

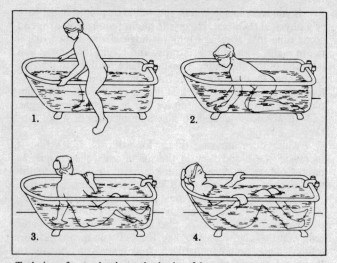

Technique for getting into a bathtub safely.

minutes. So you don't get chilled, be sure the bathroom is warm, and keep a trickle of hot water running into the tub. Try to take at least one of these long baths every day.

When your body is submerged in water, it will lose as much weight as the water it displaces. Thus, if you displace ten gallons of water, you'll reduce your weight around 83 pounds. Like the astronauts circling the globe, you'll be relatively free of gravity. The key word is *free*. Your limbs can float, so that your elbows and knees no longer have to work against the weight of muscle and bone. You should notice immediately that you can move your joints more freely than you could even lying in bed. Use your time in the water to make your spine and joints move through as much motion as you can manage, given the space limitations of your bathtub. If you're like most people, this new freedom to move will buoy your spirits, too. It's nice to know the old joints still can work—even if it's only when they're under water.

One rheumatologist, who has a private practice in suburban Philadelphia, suggests to his own patients, "Exercise your lower back, knees, hips, ankles, and wrists. There isn't enough space in a bathtub to really move your shoulders or elbows. If you can manage it, consider installing a Jacuzzi to provide a soft massage. At the spa in Baden-Baden, they also have tiny jets of carbon dioxide that shoot into the tub through tiny pinholes. The CO_2 gathers on your skin, producing a wonderful, tingling sensation. When you get out you're as pink as a baby and feel like one, too. If you can't get to Baden-Baden, a very large bathtub with a whirlpool attachment will do just fine," he says.

As you take more and more baths, however, you'll find that the exercises you do in the tub pay off outside as well. The muscles and joints, couched in the water, slowly regain strength and flexibility. Each day, a bit more is accomplished. Soon you may be able to perform some motions that seemed impossibly painful and difficult. In fact, the doctor says you should feel better in a week to ten days.

California, Here We Come

Chances are, you've heard about hot tubs. Those swingin' singles in Malibu soak in them, all the while swilling Chablis. Maybe they're so embarrassingly trendy they put you off. (Besides, what would the neighbors say?) Well, function—like beauty—is in the eye of the beholder. Ignore the stereotype and what do you have? A tub full of hot water.

It's a lot bigger than a bathtub, and for a person with arthritis that's a real plus. In a bathtub, you can't swing your arms and legs through their full range of motion. In a hot tub you can. Moreover, if you have problems with your hips, knees, shoulders, or spine, the larger tub can be a godsend. You can sit on a side bench and bend your knees, maybe eventually bringing them right up to your chin, with the water carrying their full weight. You can hold on to the rim—just as you held on to the side of the pool when you were first learning to swim—and roll your spine up and down. The heat of the water will relax your joints. The size of the tub is big enough to allow a lot of therapeutic motion, yet not as big as a swimming pool where you can lose nearby support.

There are, however, two very big disadvantages to hot tubs: their cost and their size. Prices run into the thousands because they are made of quality woods like cedar, teak, or redwood. The most common size is four feet high and five feet in diameter. For that reason, they're generally situated outdoors or in a greenhouse. Mike Stachel, owner of a Pennsylvania hot-tub dealership, says they are "super-fabulous" for those with arthritis—his wife being one. They come with a whirlpool attachment to enhance their therapeutic value. Moreover, if your doctor prescribes this treatment, the cost can be listed as a medical expense on your income tax.

Or Try a Natatorium

Think about joining the local Y, gym, or health spa so you can take advantage of the indoor swimming pool (technically called a natatorium, as many old-timers recall). Not up to swimming yet? Then don't. *Walk* instead. In water up to your chest, most of your body weight will be supported for you. Holding on to the side of the pool, or better yet, a friend's hands, practice walking. You can strengthen and reeducate your muscles and joints under water—just as racehorses are retrained after an injury.

With a technique called hydrogymnastics, you can work your entire body, achieving a wide range of health benefits, from preventing muscle wasting to improving strength, balance, and coordination. The technique is not as athletically strenuous as its name implies. You simply move in water, setting your own limits. You can wear a swim belt or "water wings" if you like. You'll need a willing partner to support your back and hips so you can make circles with your legs and arms, and to hold you by the shoulders so you can do spine stretches.

The idea behind this therapy is to simply move about and have fun. As you stretch, prance, flex, and bend, you'll develop a suppleness you probably thought you'd never see again. Don't be afraid to try lots of different movements but don't overdo. If you have any doubts about whether this technique might be harmful to you, do check with your doctor.

Running Hot and Cold

If you've got RA, or osteoarthritis in your hands and/or feet, contrast baths may be just the ticket for you. With this treatment, you place your hands or feet first into hot water, then cold. Contrast baths increase blood flow to these extremities to help healing and eliminate pain. It is for these treatments that you'll need two basins or large bowls. Fill one with cold water (60°F), the other with hot (110°F). First, place your hands or feet in the hot water for 10 minutes, then the cold for 1 minute. After this initial contrast bath, continue switching from hot to cold, putting your hands or feet in the hot water for *4* minutes, then in the cold for *1* minute. Repeat this 4-minutes-to-1 treatment six times. The entire treatment should take 41 minutes.

"Baggie" Therapy for Pain

And now, the latest medical breakthrough—the *baggie!* Doctors at the Germantown Medical Center, Philadelphia, Pennsylvania, found that you can kill arthritis pain with a baggie full of ice. For people who are not helped by heat (the usual treatment), this new, somewhat arctic approach may be the answer.

At the center, 24 patients with RA applied ice treatment to their sore knees, three times a day for four weeks. At the end of the experiment, *all* patients agreed they improved. They had more pain-free movement and muscle strength. They could stand up faster and sleep better. Perhaps most important, they could cut their dosage of medicine in half.

Here's exactly how to do this treatment. Using two large baggies, fill each with six ice cubes and a quart of cold water. Put one on top of your sore knee, and the other below. Now wrap a towel around the arrangement to hold it snugly and sit tight for 20 minutes. Do this three times a day, at evenly spaced intervals. You'll probably feel a little uncomfortable because of the intense cold. But hang on, because the Germantown patients say that feeling lasts for only 5 minutes, then the anesthetic effect takes hold. At the end of the treatment, you'll feel great.

You probably noticed that the Germantown patients used a baggie on only one knee. Suppose you have arthritis in both? Well, the amazing baggie treatment produced a mysterious effect. Even though it was applied to only one knee, the patients said it made *both* knees feel better. Peter D. Utsinger, M.D., who headed up the research team, says this unexpected benefit may not be just the power of suggestion, but actually something purely physical. Here's why: One of several effects produced by the cold therapy is an upsurge in the body's level of endorphins. These are natural chemicals that circulate through the body and actually numb pain. Quite possibly, the endorphins help relieve pain in both legs and, conceivably, anywhere else in the body, too.

* * *

All of these water treatments are effective and economical. Experiment with all of them to see which work best for you. None of them will do you any harm, and one or all may do you a whole lot of good!

12

MOVING FORWARD

Nobody ever said it would be easy. But you *can* thwart arthritis. Two essential elements are the desire to be free of the disease and a willingness to commit yourself to a self-help regimen. You'll need this firm resolve at the start, when the going is tough. One of the most important therapies for recovery, you see, is exercise to help you regain strength and flexibility. And exercising with arthritis can be a real pain in the neck (and back, shoulders, hips, fingers, or knees).

"But," you may say, "when I try to exercise, my joints really hurt. Isn't pain nature's way of telling us to stop doing something harmful?" Sure enough, that old axiom is generally true. But it isn't *absolutely* true, particularly for arthritis where a little pain is your ticket to freedom. With arthritis you *must* move your joints—ideally through their full range of motion—to keep them from freezing up and to prevent muscle wasting. Sometimes that motion hurts. But most doctors agree that in order to get results, you have to push each joint just a little past the point of discomfort during a workout. Only if the pain persists for two hours or more after exercising should you think you pushed too hard.

Remember that the cartilage in a joint has only one way of getting nourishment—from synovial fluid. And the only way that fluid can enter a joint is through exercise. Certainly, not everyone who exercises can "hit the ground running" (as the politicians like to say), and that's absolutely okay. It's more important for each person to just *begin*, no matter how modest the exercise may be. In fact, even "passive" exercise (where another person or a machine provides the muscle) can make a joint healthier. According to Robert B. Salter, M.D., professor and head of orthopaedic surgery at the University of Toronto Faculty of Medicine, under certain circumstances injured joints recover better with motion than if they had been rested in a plaster cast.

The doctor tells two interesting stories. First, he recounts an experiment where laboratory animals with injured joints were divided into three groups: in group one the injured limb was put in a plaster cast, the second group was allowed to move about as they liked in their quarters, and the third recuperated with their limbs hooked up to a machine that exercised the bad joint continuously. That third treatment was not cruel. In fact, it was just the opposite. These animals started healing in only three weeks, while the group-one animals in casts never healed. In fact, they had almost total joint destruction after ten weeks.

Dr. Salter explains that without movement, the synovial membrane gradually adheres to the joint cartilage like Scotch tape. Eventually, it obscures the joint so that the cartilage cannot get nutrition and quickly begins to degenerate. "The (animal) studies clearly show the value of CPM (continuous passive motion) in the regeneration of cartilage," he says.

The doctor's next step was to develop a machine that could provide the same sort of motion for people. At this writing, ten patients with cartilage damage have undergone treatment, all with good results. The first was a teen-age girl who could barely walk when she entered the hospital. After surgery to remove adhesions from a previous injury, she was given ten days of continuous passive motion. She went on to regain full use of her knee—to the point where she has even taken up water-skiing as a hobby.

And if that's what passive exercise can do, imagine what real exercise can accomplish.

Keep in mind, too, that these exercise routines are not only good for you, they are (or soon will be) *fun!* You have lots of programs to choose from—yoga, dancing, stretching, sports, and more. The kind you choose depends more on your personality than on what kind of arthritis you have. What you want to aim for are exercises to maintain or improve *flexibility,* exercises to increase the *strength* of the joints' surrounding muscles so you don't need external support aids, and exercises that increase your *endurance*.

Free and Easy

Let's begin at the beginning—by testing each arthritic joint to see what it can do. Say your problem is in the neck. Test it by moving your head up and down, looking as far to the right and left as you can, and rolling your head by making an imaginary circle with your chin. (If you want a nice surprise later, jot down your findings and tape them to the back of a calendar page six months from now. Your scrawled "couldn't raise arm to shoulder level" may give you quite a lift when you see how far you've come.)

After testing the joints, s-t-r-e-t-c-h them to increase their flexibility. Work with the three or four joints you feel are most important. Do all stretching exercises slowly and with care. Stretch each joint three to ten times, repeating this routine two to four times a day. If your arthritis is bad, begin at the most modest level: three stretches for each joint, twice a day. You can slowly increase the number of stretches you do.

A word of *caution:* Do *not* use painkillers when you are exercising. They too easily mask the pain, so that you can unwittingly damage a joint by pushing it too fast or too hard.

There is a feline art to stretching. The motion is languid and fluid and soft. It is *not* throwing your arms above your head and bouncing down to touch your toes. Nor is it moving to the rhythm of "hut-two-three-four." You might, however, enjoy stretching to the music of *Swan Lake* or a tune by Duke Ellington.

Ben E. Benjamin, Ph.D., author of the book, *Sports without Pain* (Summit Books, 1979), emphasizes that the best way to stretch is to ease yourself into the position. Stretching is a gentle, conditioning exercise. Relaxation is very important. Once you have extended your muscles as far as they want to go, keep breathing normally, and hold the position for 10 to 15 seconds. Next time you might stretch farther and hold the position longer.

"You must be able to tell where the action is happening," Dr. Benjamin writes. "Pay attention to precisely where the pulling sensation is. You should feel the pull in the meaty part of the muscle. If the sensation is felt near a joint only, you are stretching the ligament or tendon. Always try to do the exercise so that you feel it throughout the bulk of the muscle." Here are some stretches you can try.

SIDE STRETCH

Sit in a chair with your feet about a foot apart, and bend your body to the right, imagining as you do so that you are lifting upward against the bend. Don't hold this stretch, just repeat on the left side, then go back to the right. Try to bend five times on each side.

BACK STRETCH

Sit in the same position in an armless chair. Bend forward, bringing your arms and shoulders between your knees. Lean forward as if you were going to put your elbows on the floor. Repeat this stretch several times, and gradually build up your holding time.

NECK STRETCH

While either sitting or standing, clasp your hands behind your neck and let your head drop forward. Hold that position for 10 to 15 seconds, then raise your head and rest. Repeat the stretch, only this time, hold your hands an inch higher at the base of your skull. That is the maximum stretch and should only be done if it is comfortable.

Yoga Stretches

A comprehensive program for your neck, spine, shoulders, arms, and legs can be found in the traditional Eastern stretch routine: yoga. As a personal form of exercise, it can be individually tailored to fit your needs. Just listen to your body's language. It will tell you where you need the most stretch and when to stop short of strain. "Never exceed your body's capabilities" is the first commandment of yoga, and that includes capabilities which have been hampered by arthritis.

A Back Rest

Exercise and rest are both important to anyone with arthritis. But if you have bad back pain, it may be almost impossible to find a position that's comfortable enough to *let* you rest.

Sandy Burkhart, Ph.D., comes to the rescue. An associate professor of anatomy at West Virginia University, and practicing physical therapist, he recommends a rest position that eases acute back pain.

Place an armless chair where you will have room to lie down beside it. Then, put some pillows on the floor approximately where your head will be. Lie down, arranging the pillows under your neck and shoulders to cushion the upper spine. Place your lower legs—from knee to heel—on the seat of the chair. If necessary, ask someone to help you lift your legs. This position reduces the curve in the small of the back. Dr. Burkart says it is very comfortable and effective in relaxing the entire spine.

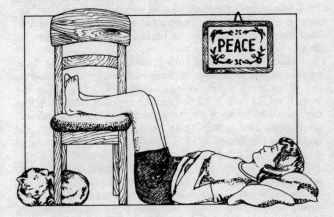

Paulynne Bennett, a woman who defeated her arthritis pain with yoga (at the age of 60!), tells of her accomplishment.

"I had all the classic symptoms of arthritis—pain and stiffness in my joints and tingling sensations, like electric currents, radiating down the entire length of my arm," recalls Paulynne. "It got so bad that I couldn't do anything comfortably, not even rest my arm on a pillow. But that was three years ago. Look at me today," she smiles, while swinging her "bad" arm back and forth like a pendulum. "My arm is perfect—thanks to yoga."

Before putting her efforts into yoga, however, Paulynne went the usual arthritis route. She visited her doctor and had X rays taken which confirmed that she had osteoarthritis in her left arm and degeneration of the spinal column. Then she embarked on a prescribed course of therapy which included taking aspirin to relieve the pain and reduce the inflammation.

"The only problem was, I ended up taking at least 6 aspirin a day," she sighs. "And some days were so bad I took 10 or 12."

Like so many others puzzled by arthritis misery, Paulynne eventually realized that she couldn't find the answer in a pill. But unlike most other 60-year-olds, she had an excellent alternative right in her living room—an exercise mat.

"I had been teaching yoga at the time of my illness," she explains. "But with all my talking and instructing and worrying about other people's yoga needs, I was neglecting my own. It wasn't until the arthritis flared up that I took stock of my own well-being. I started a personal yoga program and concentrated on loosening up the joints of my left arm and improving the flexibility of my spine. Now my joints are as flexible as they were ten years ago. It's a miracle!"

Indeed, anyone who is fighting the uphill battle against arthritis would agree that her recovery was quite a feat. But on the other hand, why should it be so surprising that yoga struck the winning blow? After all, it is an excellent form of stretching exercise. Its slow-motion movements and gentle holds reach deep into troubled joints. In addition, the easy stretches in conjunction with deep-breathing exercises relieve the tension which binds up the muscle and further tightens the joints. Yoga is exercise and relaxation rolled into one—the perfect antiarthritis formula.

Yoga is special in another way, too. It seems that a major problem in prescribing exercise is in getting the patient to follow through. If an exercise program is painful and too strenuous, it isn't likely to be continued. But yoga eases you into exercise without pain and strain. Even if you are able to move only an inch and hold a position for five seconds, you are already enhancing your body's flexibility.

Some physicians have long recognized the advantages of yogalike exercises. One is Morris A. Bowie, M.D., recently retired from Bryn Mawr Hospital and the Hospital of the University of Pennsylvania in Philadelphia. He recommends the pendulum, an arm-swinging exercise "devised by an orthopedic surgeon," for bursitis and shoulder stiffness. He also favors deep-breathing exercises for those with ankylosing spondylitis to keep the rib cage and spine flexible.

Paulynne, too, has learned of physicians who advocate such exercises. "A doctor's wife approached me after class one day and said, 'My husband prescribes this type of exercise to his patients, but he doesn't call it yoga,'" Paulynne recalls.

In fact, she can recount hundreds of similar stories. "I remember one woman I had in class who was so crippled with arthritis that it hurt me just to watch her. The first day of the course we did a simple leg pull. Sitting erect with legs outstretched, you are supposed to grasp the furthest possible point on your legs, and with elbows out, gently pull your body toward your knees. Well, this woman was in such a bad way that she could just about grasp her thighs. She could barely budge an inch.

"But she didn't let her arthritis get her down. My goodness, no. Do you know that after about six months she was able to take hold of her ankles and pull her body down till her forehead touched her knees. That's something that even people without arthritis can't do!"

It just goes to show you that a little time and a lot of perseverance can help you regain an extraordinary degree of flexibility. "But don't rush it," Paulynne warns. Begin by moving only a few inches in any exercise—until you feel

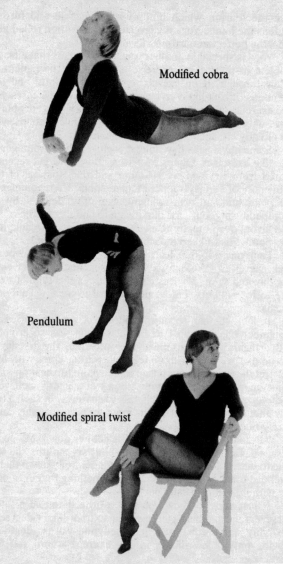

Modified cobra

Pendulum

Modified spiral twist

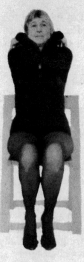

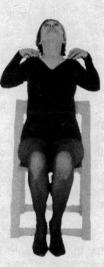

Neck and shoulder stretch

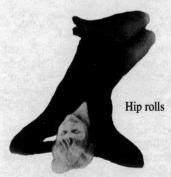

Hip rolls

slight discomfort. Then hold for a count of five. Try to repeat the same movement two or three times. Each day, try to move only an inch or so farther and hold for a second longer.

FOR THE FINGERS

Try the *flower*. Whenever you think of it, make a tight fist and hold for five seconds. Then release and stretch your hand open as far as you can for an additional five seconds. Your hand should resemble the slow-motion opening of a rose.

FOR THE SPINE

The *modified cobra* can help the entire spinal column. Lie face down on a bed or carpeted floor. With hands in front of your chest, slowly and cautiously push your torso off the floor. Raise up only a moderate distance at first and hold for five to ten seconds before slowly lowering. Eventually, you may be able to straighten out the elbows completely and tilt the head back.

FOR THE SHOULDERS

Try the *pendulum*. Leaning from the waist, with legs comfortably apart and hand on hip, slowly swing your free arm down toward the floor and up again in front of your other shoulder. After a few easy movements, repeat with your other arm.

FOR THE NECK AND UPPER BACK

Do the *modified spiral twist*. Just cross your legs (left over right) and twist your torso toward the left. Rest your right hand on your right knee, and look over your left shoulder. This position will help to give your spine a good spiral twist. Hold for five seconds. Then repeat—right leg over left, twist torso right.

Do the *neck and shoulder stretch*. Sit tall in a straight-back chair and place your fingertips on your shoulders. Slowly draw your elbows together, or in that direction. Hold for five seconds. Now move the elbows apart and back while slowly tilting your head back as far as is comfortable. Feel those shoulder blades pressing together? Hold for five seconds.

FOR THE HIPS AND LOWER SPINE

Simple *hip rolls* can increase flexibility. Lie down on a bed with your knees bent and your hands clasped under your neck. Gently twist your hips to the right as far as possible without lifting your shoulders from the bed. Hold for five seconds and then return to the starting position. Now, slowly twist to the left and hold for the same. Does your left knee touch the bed? If not, don't rush it. It will in time.

Do any or all of these yoga stretches if you can. Go at your own pace, moving slowly and gently. This ancient art may be the key to continued mobility.

That Rhythmic ROM-ba Beat

Drop the disco, bench the boogie, and chuck the cha-cha-cha. The latest dance craze—at least for those with joint disease—is called the ROM. (The letters stand for range of motion.) Developed at St. Mary's Hospital Medical Center in Madison, Wisconsin, by Diane Harlowe, director of occupational therapy and speech services, and Patricia Beadles Yu, health educator, the dance is based on the motions of the ancient Chinese exercise T'ai Chi Chuan.

You may recall seeing news broadcasts from China that show individuals stepping out on a bright morning to join their neighbors in a park or street, to do a precise set of exercises. Even the very old participate in the gentle but invigorating motions that mimic the martial gestures of attack and defense.

"We based the dance on T'ai Chi because all the movements are slow and relaxed, and each has its own meaning," explains Harlowe. They're done to a poem that presents lovely, visual images. The primary function of the dance is to help the body maintain range of motion. Most people find it an excellent way to limber up. It doesn't emphasize working any one particular joint, but if an individual wants to do that, he can alter the pattern to suit his needs. "The dance lasts only seven minutes and should be done once a day. We present it at a local health center in an eight-week session. It can be part of an overall treatment that can feature other physical therapies, and is meant to enhance but not replace them," Harlowe explains.

One of the major benefits of the dance is that it helps people get through a rather boring set of exercises where they slowly move each joint up, down, and around, as far as it will go. And if the dance makes the exercises less boring and more enjoyable, chances are they'll be done more often.

If the idea of a range-of-motion dance appeals to you, consider developing your own. Harlowe's version has you spending the day at the beach—wriggling your feet in the water (exercising the ankles), bending to scoop water (for the spine), kicking imaginary ripples (knees and hips), and so

---

EXERCISING THE TENNIS ELBOW

In some cases, arthritis is actually caused by a sport. The classic example is tennis elbow, where the tendons of the joint (rather than the cartilage) become injured. The muscle in the forearm is usually strained as well.

A player who hits with his wrists, who uses a racquet that's too tightly strung, or who hits heavy-duty balls is the most likely candidate for tennis elbow. The injury comes about when the force of the ball hitting the racquet is greater than the strength of the arm muscle.

The first step in recovery is to give up the game for as long as your elbow is sore. While the tendons are healing, work on strengthening the forearm muscle with a five-pound dumbbell. Rest your forearm on a table beside your chair, with the wrist extending over the edge. Dumbbell in hand, slowly raise and lower the weight ten times. Rest one minute, then do ten more lifts. Repeat once more.

As the exercise becomes easier, you can increase the weight of the dumbbell. When your elbow stops hurting, you're ready for the courts again.

forth. You can create your own poem so each line brings to mind a certain set of movements. It's a wonderfully creative exercise. And it's fun.

Advice for Both Rookie and Pro

Let's not overlook the benefit of athletics. Remember, all cases of arthritis are not "created equal." Some people suffer with severe disability while others, also diagnosed as having arthritis, may feel just an occasional twinge in a single joint. To overcome this disease, you have to give 100 percent. For some, that full effort means gentle exercises done in warm water. But for those with just a wince-and-twinge case, it means strenuous exercise.

"A person with arthritis may have to give up running, but he can still walk," says George Ehrlich, M.D., director of the Arthritis Center at Philadelphia's Albert Einstein Medical Center. He stresses that not everyone can do the same kind of exercise, but that everyone should exercise. His cautionary advice: Don't exercise cold, don't exercise incorrectly, don't exercise when your joints are inflamed, and don't overtax the joints.

The idea behind strenuous exercise is to get a good workout without harming yourself.

- *Swimming* is high on the list of recommended activities, particularly if you have arthritis in the weight-bearing joints. If swimming is your *modus operandi,* do it every day. Add laps as you are able. Remember to take a minute of rest every few laps.

- *Walking* is an excellent aerobic activity. It will improve your circulation, work out your heart, burn off some calories, and strengthen your muscles. Be sure to wear shoes with a good fit and flexible soles that allow your feet to bend naturally. Start with a short, easy ramble around the neighborhood and slowly increase both your pace and distance.

- *Jogging and running* are beyond the capacity of many with arthritis. However, if you have a very

POOL YOUR RESOURCES

When you are ready to exercise on your own, head for the pool with a comprehensive plan already in mind. For example, if you have trouble with your knees or feet, work out a series of progressively more difficult exercises to help those specific joints. One such series might involve standing in waist-deep water, holding on to the side of the pool. In that position, stand on one foot while rotating the ankle of your free leg. Turn your foot slowly clockwise and counterclockwise, repeating the movement several times. Then, switch feet.

Add to this basic exercise as soon as you feel ready. For instance, you might follow the ankle rotation by standing on tip-toe, then at rest. First, work with both feet together, then each separately. Eventually, you can work up to small kicks, knee-bends, and even full leg-swings.

As you grow stronger and more confident, you can create a series that works your entire body. Such a program was developed by Susan Klein, a young woman with rheumatoid arthritis. "I worked up an aquatic program in cooperation with the Metropolitan Washington Chapter of the Arthritis Foundation, which has now been adopted nationwide. It's appropriate for all age groups and any of the more than 100 different types of arthritis.

"It's a program that helps mobilize the joints, helps them gain strength, and hopefully prevents deformity. For the first 15 minutes, people just get used to being in the water—which, by the way, should never be below 82°F. Then, we spend a half hour doing range-of-motion exercises. These are much easier when performed in water. I tell the participants to use pain as a guideline. Basically, there are two kinds of pain you can experience in this program—one is from stress on a joint, the other is from unused muscle groups. If an exercise really hurts, you have to modify it. Sometimes it takes a while for long-unused muscles to get back in shape. After the exercises, we spend the last 15 minutes in the whirlpool, where the water temperature should never be above 110°F. The participants are told never to stay in the whirlpool longer than 15 minutes.

"The swimming pool is a great place for people with arthritis to socialize. It is a time to share accomplishments, fears, and frustrations, and know you are not the only one facing the challenge that arthritis offers you. This program can be adapted for both people who are good swimmers and those who can't swim at all. I use kickboards, beach balls, and Styrofoam barbells as swimming aids.

"Ironically, I'm one of the sickest people in the group. When I have a flare-up, I instruct from the pool deck—but that's not too often. I've found that we all help each other. In fact, we've formed a support group—a kind of sharing time when we can lend a shoulder to each other.

"The program has been very successful—in many ways. One of the people in the group is a woman of 29 who developed rheumatoid arthritis when she was pregnant. She fell into a serious depression. In fact, she became one of the 'behind-the-door' arthritics who was quite hostile and bitter toward her disease. Somehow she heard about my aquatic program and came to watch. Well, she got hooked on it. She's been working with us for only ten weeks, and her attitude has really turned around. She's ready to job hunt, and she's even talking about having another baby.

"I reached out my hand to her and she took it," says Susan.

mild case, and if it is limited to the joints in the upper body, this exercise may be possible. Check with your doctor first. The primary consideration in running and jogging is to avoid pounding your joints. Be sure to wear properly fitted running shoes with a cushioned sole. Jog or run only on even surfaces that "give"—like a cinder track, grass, or dirt, but *not* a sidewalk. And listen to your body.

• *Competitive sports* need doctor's approval, too. However, if tennis or racquetball is too strenuous for you, maybe you can trade down to a sport that's not as hard on the wrist, elbow, and shoulder—like badminton. It's of enormous benefit to the spirit to *play*. It proves that, yes, you can still have fun, even if you also have arthritis.

13

FOLK REMEDIES

Here's an old Pennsylvania Dutch cure for warts: Cut a potato in half and rub the white part against your warts while standing with your back to a full moon. When you've rubbed enough, throw the potato over your shoulder.

Generations of Pennsylvania Dutch have removed their warts with this peculiar little treatment, just as they have treated their upset stomachs with catnip tea and their chest colds with a rub of goose grease. Most medical doctors would smile with warm amusement, saying that if the treatment worked, it would be, in fact, the result of the placebo effect (where your mind does the curing because of a profound belief in the treatment).

But suppose some years from now medical science discovers an as yet unknown enzyme or alkaloid in the potato that does in fact (and not in mind) dissolve warts. Who then would smile with amusement—the clear-skinned Pennsylvanian or the lab-bound scientist?

The point to be made is that remedies are passed down through generations because they *do* work. Maybe science can't explain *why,* but that alone is not reason enough for dismissing them out of hand as sheer quackery. Sometimes science finally catches up to folk wisdom, adding credence to a treatment that a knowing grandma has been recommending all along. Examples abound.

One folk cure involved boiling the bark of the willow tree in a small amount of water. Drinking this brew was said to relieve pain. And in fact, in 1827, the French chemist Leroux extracted a painkilling substance. He named it salicin, after the willow genus *salix*. Today, that substance is the basis of the most commonly used drug in the world: aspirin.

In India, farmers and peasants used the snake plant *(Rauwolfia serpentina)* to settle their nerves. It later became the basis for the world's first tranquilizer. And in hot climates, local residents depended on the bark of the cinchona tree to provide relief from malaria. Today, the concoction made from that bark goes by the name quinine. Likewise, the historic use of the foxglove plant for heart ailments led to the common cardiac prescription drug, digitalis.

Keep all these examples of folk wisdom in mind as you read the following remedies for arthritis. Many people swear by them. And some are being scientifically verified as you read these words.

Copper vs. Arthritis Pain

Most doctors say they're plain silly, the Arthritis Foundation thinks they're the crown jewels of quackery, but chemist W. Ray Walker, Ph.D., knows how copper bracelets work to calm arthritis pain and inflammation.

To provide an understanding for Dr. Walker's experiments that led to his fascinating discovery, let's take a quick look at the role of copper in the body. It was determined to be essential for health in 1928. It is necessary for normal metabolism, and for the development and continued health of normal tissues. Therefore, it may be required for the prevention of arthritis. But copper cannot be synthesized in the body, and therefore it must be supplied by outside sources—usually the diet.

Now here's where Dr. Walker's discovery becomes exciting. This chemist from the University of Newcastle, New South Wales, Australia, was thoroughly skeptical about the effectiveness of copper bracelets. However, he conducted several clinical tests of copper jewelry to find out if maybe, just maybe, there was something to this folk remedy. He began quite simply by asking a group of 23 arthritics who had previously worn copper bracelets to switch to aluminum. More than half reported that they didn't feel nearly as well wearing their new bracelets.

Another group was asked to try copper bracelets for a month, and many reported a noticeable improvement. And finally, a group of 40 copper bracelet wearers were asked to forgo their bracelets for two months: 14 couldn't go the distance.

"Previous users are significantly worse when not wearing their bracelets," Dr. Walker writes in the journal *Agents and Actions*.

So, the doctor could see that for some reason the bracelets work. But why and how? Clearly they're not magical, like Wonder Woman's wristlets. Perhaps the copper somehow can enter the body through the skin to perform its wonders.

Perhaps. Thus, Dr. Walker examined the bracelets and found that each lost an average of 13 milligrams of copper per month—dissolved by the sweat of the wearer. And finally, conclusively, the doctor had a biopsy done on tissue removed from a finger on which he wore a copper ring. And there, even to incredulous eyes, was the characteristic blue stain— more than skin deep.

Dr. Walker reasoned that copper can move through the skin, into the bloodstream, and then presumably to the liver, where it can be readied for action. Spurred by his theory and the remarkable results of his experiments, he's currently developing a copper-based lotion. When applied to the skin over an affected joint, he hopes the compound will allow the mineral quick and sure access to inflamed tissue.

Dr. Walker's verification of copper's powers is not alone. Biochemist Helmar Dollwet, Ph.D., working at the University of Akron, in Ohio, has also investigated the properties of these bracelets. "My research indicates that copper from a bracelet reacts with chemicals within perspiration, dissolves, and is then absorbed through the skin and circulated through the bloodstream to the afflicted area. It is the copper . . . which exerts a beneficial role when inside the affected joint. The role of the copper itself is very new to this research and something we are continuing to study," he said. "Based on these new findings, I think it would be appropriate for the medical profession to reconsider the validity of the copper bracelet in the treatment of arthritis," he recommended.

Perhaps that is the *how* of copper bracelets, but what about the *why*? Some doctors and scientists speculate that the average person may have a copper deficiency, which may be remedied by the absorption of copper through the skin.

"I don't think most diets are sufficient in copper," says Leslie M. Klevay, M.D., of the USDA's Human Nutrition Laboratory in North Dakota. "Unfortunately, 84 percent of the diets we've examined yield less than 1.67 milligrams. (Two milligrams is the suggested daily requirement.) What's more, the copper content of food seems to be declining." The amount of copper available in any food—plant or animal—depends on the soil on which it was raised. And we have seen severe soil depletion in this country in recent years.

Might a possible copper deficiency cause or aggravate rheumatoid arthritis (RA)?

"Rheumatoid arthritis appears to be a relatively recent disease," says Kim Rainsford, Ph.D., a chemical pathologist at King's College Hospital Medical School in London. In the last hundred years, it's become all too common throughout our population but, he notes, "in Europe in the Middle Ages, it seemed that the poorer people—and remember, they used copper utensils for cooking—were less likely to get the disease." Presumably, a healthy dose of the mineral found its way into their food.

Interestingly, he relates, copper miners also are relatively arthritis-proof. "Now we know that there are changes in the protective status of the immune system in copper-deficient states and it's a well-known fact that cadmium, lead, and other toxic heavy metals present in the modern environment work against the beneficial action of copper," says Dr. Rainsford.

Swearing by Fish Oil

Tom Mealey, a burly 69-year-old Californian, gave up his copper bracelet ("which worked okay but it turned my arm green") for a daily dose of cod-liver oil. "I found out about it from a man who does my yard work. One day he asked me, 'Tom, why are you limping?' and I told him I'd broken my hip and now I have arthritis in my leg.

" 'Well,' he says, 'why don't you do what I do and take cod-liver oil?' So I started, and it took about two months before I began to feel better. But then I began to feel *a lot* better. Now I don't go a day without taking my capsules. If I forget for any length of time—two or three weeks, for example—I can hardly walk on my leg," says Mealey. And in the true spirit of all folk remedies, he passed along the same advice he got from the yard man to an elderly neighbor with a bent spine. "She can't straighten her back, but at least her pain is gone," he recounts.

In this case, the reason why this folk remedy works is no mystery at all. Cod-liver oil is loaded with vitamin D, a nutritional must for our bones. This vitamin makes sure that calcium is available to be deposited in the bones by allowing our intestine to absorb it better. In fact, if we get enough vitamin D in our diets, the amount of calcium absorbed by the intestine can *triple*. The Recommended Dietary Allowance (RDA) is 400 International Units (I.U.), provided mostly by vitamin D–enriched milk.

Cod-liver oil has long been a standard folk remedy for arthritis, and vitamin D therapy has been used in the past as a treatment for certain bone diseases. Somewhere along the line—probably with the advent of steroids—cod-liver oil was almost forgotten. Too bad, really, because in addition to personal recommendations, its use has been supported by medical tests.

In a study done years ago at the Brusch Medical Center in Cambridge, Massachusetts, 98 people with arthritis were treated with cod-liver oil, but in a very special way. They had to take it first thing in the morning on an empty stomach, and then restrict their fluid intake throughout the rest of the day.

The results were remarkable. Fully 93 percent showed major improvement and 90 percent showed favorable changes in blood chemistry. The blood sedimentation rates (which measure the severity of inflammation) dropped consistently from averages of 20 to 30 down to 0 to 12 within a period of two to five months.

The patients were a mixed group, some suffering with RA, others with osteoarthritis, and some with gout. Many had been the route of arthritis therapy—steroids, hormones, gold salts, paraffin wax baths, aspirin, and even physiotherapy—all without success. But after as short a time as 2 weeks (the longest was 20), these people experienced a marked reduction of pain. They had less fatigue, less swelling, better mobility, and generally felt better all around.

The RDA for vitamin D is 400 I.U. daily. You can get vitamin D naturally from sunlight, or from certain foods—primarily fish oil, egg yolk, milk, and butter. (Most milk in the United States is fortified with additional vitamin D.) Therefore, it's not too difficult to get an adequate dose of the vitamin, that is, provided you get out in the sunshine and drink your milk. For many of us, however, it is more convenient and reliable to supplement our diets with cod-liver oil capsules.

Be aware, however, that the law of diminishing returns applies to vitamin D. Levels above 1,800 I.U. a day seem to work against calcium intake and, because the vitamin can be stored and accumulated in the body, the danger of toxicity does exist.

Alfalfa and Arthritis

Robert Fickardt of Torrance, California, says his doctor pooh-poohed the idea of alfalfa as an arthritis treatment. "He said, 'Won't do you any good but probably won't hurt you any—so if it eases your mind, go ahead and take it.' Well, my wife had arthritis in her hands and wrists, and she swears that alfalfa tablets have eased the pain and allowed her to use her hands again.

"Betty and I have been taking the tablets for seven years, and we're about as free from aches and pains as people our ages can expect to be. Neither of us has a sign of the arthritis that once plagued us both.

"We are aware that the arthritis would probably have disappeared even if we had not continued taking alfalfa tablets. However, we both take our six tablets religiously every morning. We are just not taking any chances," says Fickardt.

Does this leafy legume have some magical hold over arthritis pain? If it does, it's yet to be proven by science. But many, many people like the Fickardts rely on alfalfa for pain relief. Some take tablets while others rely on a pungent brew of tea.

If you'd like to try this unusual drink, here's how to prepare it. Cook but do not boil one ounce of alfalfa seeds (those sold for sprouting are best) in 1¼ pints of water. Use a glass or enamel pan. Keep the water moving for half an hour. Then strain and squeeze the seeds to extract more fluid. Cool and refrigerate the tea but do not store it for more than 24 hours. To use, mix the strong base with an equal amount of water. Add honey, if you like. Take six or seven cups or four or five glasses a day for at least two weeks.

Cherries for Gout

Cherries for epilepsy, said a physician of ancient Greece. Cherries for scarlet fever, claimed rural folk doctors. And, wrote an herbalist, cherries for gout. The herbalist described how a person with gout cured himself by "taking eight cherries at each change of the moon."

Ludwig Blau, Ph.D., must have had a more stubborn case of gout because he upped the recommendation to six to eight cherries each day. He didn't get the idea from an herbalist, though. Looking for something to eat one evening, he snacked on a bowl of cherries. The next day, the pain in his gouty big toe—pain so intense he used a wheelchair—was gone. And it never came back as long as he ate cherries. But if he gave them up for even a few days, the gout returned.

This information was printed in an early edition of *Prevention* magazine, eliciting a number of letters. Many readers wrote to say they too have successfully treated their gout with cherries. A man who suffered with gout for 15 years got almost total relief. A woman whose gouty, swollen knee ached and throbbed for 2 years cured herself in a week by eating cherries. Canned, frozen, or fresh do the trick, readers say. And it doesn't matter if they are the sweet or sour variety.

And once your gout has cleared up, life can be just a bowl of you-know-what!

The Sting!

Among the more unconventional folk therapies is one that sounds absolutely painful—bee stings. And we're talking about hundreds upon hundreds of them, not merely one or two welts. Yet this old folk therapy has many enthusiastic followers who tell anyone who'll listen that bee stings relieve arthritis pain, sometimes for good.

The rumor has been kicking around for centuries that people who keep bees (and presumably are stung frequently) never get arthritis. Some ancient physicians accepted the notion that bee stings could even prevent arthritis from developing. What could bee venom contain that gives it these marvelous curative powers?

According to Joseph Broadman, M.D., in his book *Bee Venom* (G. P. Putnam's Sons, 1962), the substance itself is "a water-clear liquid with a sharp, bitter taste and an aromatic odor comparable to bananas." Analysis shows it contains two proteins—mellitin and apamine—that cause the pituitary and adrenal glands to produce more cortisone. This hormone is an effective and dramatic anti-inflammatory substance that is often prescribed by doctors to reduce pain and swelling. It's important to note, however, that cortisone produced naturally in your own body does not create the devastating side effects of artificial cortisone. (More about that in chapter 15.) Thus, it seems there is a sound scientific basis for this old remedy, too.

Studies by Major James Vick, a scientist at Walter Reed Hospital, showed that these high cortisone levels could be maintained for several days after an injection of bee venom. Working with arthritic dogs, Vick spaced the injections carefully and measured an increased cortisone output for almost four months. During this time, the dogs' mobility *tripled*.

Some old-timers rely on live bees for their treatments. Using long tweezers, they place a bee against the sore joint and let him sting. They repeat these stings, building up to as many as 60 or more a day. Others prefer to use an injectible form, the result of the work of Allen W. Benton and others at Cornell University in Ithaca, New York. They gather pure venom from bees who land on a length of clear plastic wrap stretched over an electrically charged grid. When the insects settle down, they get a small shock which—you guessed it— causes them to sting the plastic. The venom drips through the hole made by the stinger and collects on its underside. The lucky bees usually can extract themselves unharmed, living to sting another day. By the way, it takes 50,000 bees to produce one gram of pure venom.

If you are interested in trying this therapy, you *absolutely must* be tested first for an allergy to bee stings.

The Latest Folk Remedy: DMSO

You've probably seen the signs in flea markets, drugstores, and even gas stations: "We have DMSO." Or maybe you read about it in magazines such as *Sports Illustrated*, where they call it *eau de sport* and describe how world-class athletes like Alberto Salazar use it on sprains and strains. Or maybe you learned about it from the television show "60 Minutes"? What is this stuff? And, more important, how safe is it?

The letters DMSO stand for dimethyl sulfoxide, a by-product of wood pulp manufacture. It has been around for years, used as a paint thinner, an additive to chemical products, and as a solvent. In the late 1950s, the Crown Zellerbach Paper Company asked one of its chemists, Robert Herschler, to find another profitable use for this by-product. As he worked with it, one of the first things he noticed was its "carrier effect"—that is, its ability to move a second substance along with it through a membrane. Initially, he was working with plants, hoping to develop a way that DMSO could move fungicides and antibiotics from the outside into the circulatory system of the plants. One day, working in his lab at home, he burned his hand with a chemical. In a book about him, he is quoted as saying:

> Blisters erupted. The skin became inflamed. "I reached for the DMSO," Herschler remembers, "because I knew it could draw water away from the blisters. What astonished me was that the pain disappeared within minutes, and so did the blisters."
>
> *DMSO: The True Story of a Remarkable Pain-Killing Drug,* by Barry Tarshis (William Morrow and Co., 1981)

Herschler soon met Stanley Jacob, a surgeon. Together they began to explore DMSO's medical potential. Before long they had tried it on cold sores, sprains, burns, and arthritis. The two were extremely enthusiastic about the results.

But the story so far does not have a happy ending. The use of DMSO is surrounded by controversy. It has been approved for treating only one condition, a rare and painful bladder disease called interstitial cystitis. Otherwise, it has been banned for use as a medicine since 1965 because studies showed it caused eye damage in laboratory animals.

At this writing, even the one approved use is in jeopardy. Dr. Jacob has been indicted by a federal grand jury in Maryland for allegedly bribing the Food and Drug Administration (FDA) official who recommended DMSO for the treatment of interstitial cystitis. Both men have pleaded not guilty.

The indictment says the payments, totaling more than $30,000, were made "for and because of official acts performed or to be performed" by the FDA medical officer. But supporters of Dr. Jacob say the money was a loan to help pay the costs incurred by the officer's wife, who was dying from a chronic disease.

In the meantime—with or without FDA approval—DMSO is being used daily by uncounted throngs of people. They rely on it to reduce pain and swelling, and swear the stuff works. Most use it just like a liniment or lotion, swabbing it over a sore spot and letting it sink in. Within minutes, they experience a taste in the mouth usually described as being like raw oysters. They also develop telltale DMSO breath—which, it's rumored, can drop an ox in its tracks.

Once the DMSO has soaked in, it takes only minutes for it to enter the bloodstream. It is drawn to water, like a magnet. It hurries to any swollen spots in the body, latching on to the blood, lymph fluid, or pus that has collected there, moving into the bloodstream for disposal. Once the liquid is gone from the sore spot, so is the swelling and much of the pain.

Sounds good, right? Unfortunately, there are a few wrinkles to iron out. For example, you remember the "carrier effect" that got Herschler so excited? Well, that same ability to carry molecules along can result in DMSO carrying pollutants, pesticides, who-knows-what right into the blood of a user's body. The problem is compounded by the fact that DMSO is totally unregulated, so that the bottle you pick up at the flea market may contain traces of just about anything in the DMSO.

Furthermore, DMSO comes in various strengths—50 percent, 90 percent, and 100 percent. Even its most enthusiastic supporters, Herschler and Dr. Jacob, don't recommend using the stuff sold on the street. In the book, *DMSO: The True Story of a Remarkable Pain-Killing Drug* (written by Barry Tarshis, from information supplied by Herschler and Dr. Jacob), they caution, "Make certain the DMSO is pure. This is not easy to do since nearly all the DMSO sold on the black market today is commercial-grade DMSO and could conceivably carry impurities that might cause adverse reactions." The Arthritis Foundation's Dr. Frederic C. McDuffie adds that the 90 percent solution is the kind used by veterinarians, and the 100 percent DMSO is an industrial solvent. Since neither type is meant to be used by people, he warns that they're not manufactured to the degree of purity required for a medication.

Let's take a look at a random bottle of DMSO, purchased at a local drugstore. The label reads:

Product #507 (pharmaceutical grade)
DMSO/ 90% pure / no acetone solvent
Note: This product is intended to be used as a
solvent only. The choice of the process used in
various forms of applications of this product are
[sic] the sole responsibility of the customer.

Here's what the label says on the back of the bottle:

KEEP OUT OF THE REACH OF CHILDREN.
Not to be used internally. Rubber gloves should be
worn while using. Avoid skin contact. DMSO is a
potent solvent and may have a deleterious effect on
fabrics, plastics, and other materials. In the event of
a local reaction such as burning or smarting sensation, flush the skin with water and consult a physician immediately.

Avoid skin contact? Wear rubber gloves? What's going on here? According to Herschler's and Dr. Jacob's book, no one should use DMSO stronger than 70 percent. If the stuff you have is stronger, they recommend diluting it with water until you achieve 70 percent. They also suggest that you do not use it every day. "Clinical experience shows that DMSO works best when you go off it for a day or so every now and then. One of the schedules that some chronic pain sufferers follow is to use DMSO for five days and then to go off it on the weekend," their book says.

As anyone can plainly see, trying to use DMSO safely is a tricky business. Its manufacture is not regulated by the government. It is being sold willy-nilly so that a consumer doesn't know if he's buying a paint thinner or a horse rub. No scientific studies of any consequence are available to tell you exactly what the benefits or drawbacks of long-term use are. Even the label on the bottle tells you that you're strictly on your own if you use the stuff.

DMSO is not like other folk remedies which have been around for many, many years—a kind of *de facto* proof of their safety. It's a strong product that can have some serious side effects. In addition to bad breath and the danger of carrying toxic substances into the bloodstream, it's been found that intravenous use can cause severe liver damage. And, according to Brian H. Swanson, Ph.D., of Jefferson University in Philadelphia, Pennsylvania, it also can limit the effectiveness of the arthritis drug Clinoril.

People are rubbing it in, some are drinking it, and some are even injecting it—all without knowing what may happen to their health as a result. It's a dangerous treatment, whether your next-door neighbor endorses it or not.

If and when DMSO is approved, a high-quality product will be available. It also will have been studied for side effects, if any. At this writing, just one study is under way. A group of major arthritis centers has entered into a cooperative arrangement to evaluate the effect of DMSO on finger ulcers in scleroderma. Maybe this study will lead to others, so that you—as a consumer and a person with arthritis—will be able to make an educated judgment about using DMSO.

14

RELIEF FROM PAIN— WITHOUT DRUGS

Chances are, if you've had arthritis for any length of time, you're taking a drug to deaden the pain. These drugs can range from common aspirin to more sophisticated forms of aspirin like Motrin, or to heavy-duty medications like Butazolidin or cortisone. And chances are, they do give you some relief. But you've probably noticed they also have side effects, including one medical books don't mention—they drain the wallet.

In the last decade or so, a whole range of new treatments for pain has been developed. They are not drugs. Instead, they're alternative therapies that are reasonably inexpensive and have no known side effects. Used in the very best pain clinics across the country, these therapies include acupuncture, transcutaneous electrical nerve stimulation (TENS), acupressure, myotherapy, and more.

The medical establishment is only beginning to warm to these drugless treatments for pain. For one thing, doctors like to cure diseases, not just deal with the pain they cause. For another, they are not taught about them in most medical schools and therefore don't recognize them as potentially valuable therapies.

But let's face facts. Arthritis doesn't have a cure—at least not yet. It generates a lot of pain—every day for years to come. If you stick with drugs, you may end up dealing with side effects that are worse than the disease.

Keep an open mind when considering the treatments about to be discussed. Acupuncture, for instance, has been around for thousands of years. The philosophy behind the treatment sounds pretty strange to Western ears, but science—in its own "show me" way—has verified that it really does work.

Pains and Needles

Acupuncture broke on the American scene like a thunderstorm in July of 1971. *New York Times* columnist James Reston was touring the People's Republic of China in one of the first waves of Westerners to wash across that newly opened border. Suddenly he was stricken with an attack of acute appendicitis and rushed to a hospital in Peking.

His appendix was removed and he was treated for postoperative pain by acupuncture. In a page-one story splashed across *The New York Times,* Reston described how an acupuncturist placed several long needles into the outer part of his right elbow and below each knee, somehow (but *how?*) easing the pain in his gut.

Reaction among American medical professionals ran the gamut. Some thought acupuncture worked through hypnotism, others thought it was just bizarre quackery. The few doctors and health professionals who did look into the explanation offered by Chinese acupuncturists were almost immediately put off by its fairy-tale quality.

The Chinese told of meridians along which life energy called *"chi"* coursed through the body. However, meridians could become blocked. The blockage would disturb the balance of *chi,* allowing disease to develop. To reopen these channels, one had to stimulate a few points on the body—usually nowhere near the ache or pain—with hair-thin needles. The special points and meridians have fanciful names like Gate of Heaven and Heart Governor. Western medicine shrugged its collective shoulders and went back to the lab.

In the intervening years, however, it's been proven that nerve fibers do transmit a kind of *chi*—only Western doctors call it "bioelectricity." In fact, a gate theory of pain relief has been developed which proposes that if you overload certain nerve fibers with sensations other than pain—like those caused by acupuncture needles—you can block the pain message from ever reaching the brain. And work at Phila-

delphia's Albert Einstein Medical Center has shown that
these fibers transmit their messages along certain nerve net-
works that correspond with acupuncture meridians and their
points.

Additional research is being done at the University of
Southern California, where Charles K. Haun, M.D., says,
"Basically acupuncture 'needles' the nervous system." According to Dr. Haun, acupuncture apparently affects the autonomic (involuntary) portions of the nervous system, the
immune antibody system, possibly even the endocrine system, and it somehow relaxes muscles and enhances blood
circulation.

There are also a number of scientific studies which show
that acupuncture increases the amount of "endorphins," the
body's own natural painkiller. These morphinelike substances are found in the brain, the pituitary and adrenal
glands, spinal fluid, the gastrointestinal tract, and the blood.
They dramatically reduce pain.

An article in the *British Medical Journal* describes some
of these studies. In one, a rabbit was treated with acupuncture. Its cerebrospinal fluid was transferred to a second
rabbit that was not being treated. The second rabbit was
shown to be unaffected by pain. In other experiments, people
underwent acupuncture, then were given a drug called naloxone, which counteracts the analgesic effects of endorphins.
Before the naloxone, the people felt no pain. After the drug,
they did.

Eureka! We now know what the Chinese have known for
5,000 years: acupuncture works!

ACUPUNCTURE AND ARTHRITIS

And now that the West knows acupuncture's true, it's
also being tried; pain clinics and family practitioners all
across the country use the treatment successfully. Louise
Oftedal Wensel, M.D., author of the book, *Acupuncture in
Medical Practice* (Reston Publishing Co., 1980), says, "Acupuncture is the least expensive, as well as the safest and most
effective treatment for many chronic disorders. It can usually
be given on an outpatient basis. . . . Some patients, as well
as their relatives and friends, can even be taught to give

enough acupuncture or acupressure to relieve a specific type of pain without the danger or expense of drugs."

At the Maimonides Medical Center in Brooklyn, New York, doctors have been using acupuncture to wean their patients off drugs that counteract pain. "If we have to use drugs, we consider it a kind of defeat," says Philip H. Sechzer, M.D. An anesthesiologist himself, Dr. Sechzer heads a team of pain-control specialists that includes neurosurgeons, internists, psychologists, and oral surgeons. Their main goal is to prevent pain during surgery and to relieve it when it accompanies a disease such as arthritis.

Dr. Sechzer described a case of a man who had been out of work for two years with painful arthritis.

"He walked only with difficulty and with the help of a cane. During the first four acupuncture treatments, the swelling in his feet went down to the point where he was able to get his left shoe on without difficulty," he told a group attending an acupuncture convention in New York.

During the fourth to sixth treatments, the pain in his feet subsided completely but his left knee remained stiff. By the sixth and seventh treatments there was no pain—just some discomfort in the left knee, right foot, and hand.

Treatment continued and by the time the man underwent his tenth to sixteenth treatments he was well enough to return to work part-time.

The Maimonides Medical Center has been experimenting with acupuncture since late 1972 when it was still considered a new and quite unusual procedure. Since that time, much of the hoopla surrounding the treatment has subsided, leaving the field open to serious researchers who have pretty well determined how the Oriental treatment can be included in a Western medical practice.

Initial results from Maimonides indicate that acupuncture may have an important role to play in arthritis. In an article which appeared in an issue of the *Bulletin of the New York Academy of Medicine* shortly after their early studies, Dr. Sechzer and a colleague, Soon Jack Leung, M.D., compiled figures on patients who came for treatment during a six-month period. They reviewed its effect on 223 patients who received a total of 1,271 acupuncture treatments for conditions ranging from arthritis to multiple sclerosis.

The largest group of patients consisted of 109 individuals who suffered from different types of arthritis, such as rheumatoid arthritis (RA) and osteoarthritis. Final figures showed that 81 patients classified as having arthritis of one kind or another experienced either complete or partial improvement. Of the remaining patients, 27 had no improvement and 1 became worse.

On the country's other coast, doctors were discovering the very same thing. Richard Kroening, M.D., and David E. Bresler, Ph.D., then working at UCLA's Chronic Pain Clinic in Los Angeles, found that a significant number of patients—particularly the elderly with osteoarthritis aches and pains—can benefit tremendously from acupuncture therapy. No hospitalization or constant medical supervision is needed, and it is not a traumatic procedure.

One of their patients, a 67-year-old woman, had been living with generalized osteoarthritis for years. It had become especially painful in her hips and knees, making stair climbing, walking, even sleeping, almost impossible. Medication did nothing, and only heat offered a modicum of relief.

Her first 5 acupuncture treatments failed to relieve her pain, but by the sixth, she felt results. She could stand longer, walk easier, and her pain was markedly less sharp. After 13 or 14 treatments, she continued to improve and found her pain only "mild."

After six months of acupuncture, she stopped going to the clinic. Six months later, her pain returned—but not as bad as it was originally.

"We consider her a success," Dr. Bresler says. "We don't promise complete pain relief, only that we can help a great deal."

WHAT TO EXPECT

If you decide to give acupuncture a try, check the listing of pain-control clinics in Appendix 1 at the back of this book to find those that offer acupuncture. When you go for your first treatment, don't be put off by the needles. The sensation is *not* like "getting a shot." Acupuncture needles are no thicker than a whisker, and run from ½ to 4 inches in length. The depth of insertion varies, as does the length of time the needles are left in. Because they are so thin they don't cause much pain when they are inserted, and there is almost never any bleeding. Often the needles are gently rotated by hand or by very low voltage electrical attachments. In general, no more than 10 to 12 needles are used during a single acupuncture session and the number of sessions can range from 3 to over 100.

According to Dr. Wensel, the main treatment point for arthritis is located near the hip joint. Branches of nerves—including the sciatic nerve—converge in this region. Be advised that this point requires a long needle for deep insertion.

CHOOSING AN ACUPUNCTURIST

Before you let your fingers do the walking through the acupuncture listings, keep in mind that there are a lot of people practicing acupuncture—and not all of them know what they're doing. Some states have laws that acupuncture can be performed only under the direct supervision of a licensed physician. The doctor will diagnose the ailment and determine whether acupuncture is an appropriate treatment. He or she will then supervise the acupuncturist closely enough to make sure that the procedure is as germ-free as any other treatment that pricks the skin.

Do be sure a doctor diagnoses your condition before treatment. Some skilled acupuncturists do not speak English well enough to understand the subtleties of your description when you recount the nature of your complaint.

Are you a candidate for successful acupuncture treatments? According to studies at the Mayo Clinic on 172 patients with similar ages and backgrounds, you're most likely to find relief if you've had your pain for three years or less, and if you've never been operated on for pain. If, however, you feel dependent on drugs to ease you through the day, you may not find relief as easily as other candidates.

Dr. Wensel practices at the Washington Acupuncture Center, where more than 10,000 patients have been treated for various forms of arthritis. More than 80 percent have had significant improvement. In her book she explains, "Most patients have their pain, swelling, and stiffness significantly reduced by the time they have had six to ten acupuncture treatments. Some of them have remained free from these symptoms for more than five years. . . . Others have had a recurrence of pain after a year or six months, but the pain was relieved again after another course of treatment. Some people with severe rheumatoid arthritis have been able to stay almost symptom-free by having maintenance treatments once a week or less often."

Needles and TENS

There's a kind of electric aspirin called TENS, which stands for the rather unwieldy phrase, transcutaneous electrical nerve stimulation. It's a fairly new treatment that works almost the same way acupuncture does—but without needles. Instead, it uses electric current. And it, too, must be prescribed by a doctor.

When you undergo TENS treatment, you'll be given a little black box that holds a tiny, battery-operated generator. Cables run from the generator to electrodes that attach to the skin. Usually a doctor or a physical therapist fastens the electrodes—either along specific neurological pathways or right over a sore spot—and lets you control the knob that increases or decreases the intensity of the current. However, for severe cases of intractable pain, TENS electrodes can be implanted right in the body. And some athletes tape a unit to an injury so they can play even though they're hurting. In other words, there's a certain amount of flexibility to a TENS treatment.

The workings of this little machine are based on the gate theory that also explains acupuncture. Your perception of pain is blocked by an electrical signal transmitted through the skin to nerves. The electrical message also spurs the brain to produce higher than normal amounts of endorphins and other natural painkillers produced by the body. These endorphins stay in the body for hours, and in some cases, even days.

Reports of a study in Australia on the benefits of TENS therapy are very encouraging. There, 60 patients with acute and chronic pain (including arthritis) were treated with TENS. Forty percent gained *complete* relief from pain and another 28 percent had substantial relief. One patient in the study was a 74-year-old woman who had suffered with arthritis in her spine, hips, knees, and hands. Previous treatments—including anti-inflammatory drugs, diathermy, steroid injections, and more—didn't help. However, TENS did. After only four sessions she was able to walk without a cane and the very bad swelling in her knees was considerably reduced.

Another patient had arthritis in the lower back. He had been successfully treated with drugs, but his last painful episode had lasted for five months without relief. It was destroying his sleep and leaving him unable to work. When a TENS unit was attached over the sciatic nerve, he experienced an almost immediate lessening of pain. It continued to fade for two hours after the treatment, allowing him to get his first good night's sleep in months.

The one common disadvantage of using a TENS is that it causes a skin irritation. However, lots of people with arthritis are more than willing to trade their aches and pains for a skin rash.

Pressure Points and Trigger Points

Other treatments available to people with arthritis include acupressure and myotherapy. Acupressure is exactly what its name implies—pressing on the acupuncture points that normally would be pricked with a needle. The pressure can be applied with a finger, knuckle, elbow, or a small, blunt object.

Myotherapy is *not* exactly what its name implies. Rather, it means different things to different therapists. In general, the word implies some kind of treatment given to a muscle. Various pain clinics offer myotherapy through massage, ultrasound treatments, or other muscle manipulation.

However, to a very small number (29 at this writing), myotherapy is spelled with a capital letter. It's a specific course of treatment developed by Bonnie Prudden (the exercise-on-TV person) in 1976. Working as an exercise therapist, she developed corrective exercises and located trigger points—little knots of pain and stiffness in the muscles. She'd mark them and send the patient off to the doctor for an injection of a novocainelike drug right into the point. One day she accidentally discovered that by pressing a trigger point she could eliminate pain. In her book *Pain Erasure: The Bonnie Prudden Way* (M. Evans and Co., 1980), she writes, "Old traumas leave footprints all over the body." Trigger points are laid down over the years, and "the longer the trigger points related to arthritis go unattended, however, the more time the muscles have in which to learn bad habits."

She offers a training course at her School of Physical and Myotherapy in Lenox, Massachusetts, from which the first class graduated in 1981. One Bonnie Prudden-certified therapist, Nancy Bleam, of Allentown, Pennsylvania, says that myotherapy can offer some relief to those with arthritis. However, the therapy does not help the joint itself. "Arthritis sets up a pain/muscle spasm/more pain cycle. You have to break the cycle by relaxing the muscle. Then the arthritis becomes more comfortable. However, the pain often returns."

Because the relief is temporary, myotherapists like to teach the technique to a family member or close friend who can locate the trigger points and press away the pain.

An Unusual Suggestion

And here's one final recommendation for drug-free relief from arthritis pain: sex. Wanda Sadoughi, M.D., director of the Sexual Dysfunction Clinic at the Cook County Hospital in Chicago, Illinois, discovered this little tidbit of information quite by accident. "We weren't looking for this. We were studying this area in handicapped patients. It was striking that a number of these patients with arthritis found it important enough to mention. They volunteered that sex helped them, sometimes in striking ways. They'd say 'I was free of

pain for several hours thereafter.' Not 'The pain was reduced,' but 'I was *free* of pain.' The relief lasted four to six
hours.

"Ages of people in the study ranged from the twenties to
68—but mostly they were older. In some cases, the arthritis
was severe. There were some people we thought were too
crippled to be interested in sex. We found to our surprise
they were still having sex and experienced positive results,"
she says.

Why should sex make arthritis pain disappear? "There
may be an emotional component in arthritis, so that could be
a factor. Stress is both psychological and physiological—and
sex can alleviate both," Dr. Sadoughi says.

"It is also connected with self-esteem, the feeling that
you're still wanted and still worthwhile. Some patients allow
arthritis to disable them unnecessarily. Sex can affect your
entire outlook on life, making it positive rather than hope-
less."

And isn't that good news.

15

THE MANY DRUGS FOR ARTHRITIS

*The art of medicine consists of amusing the patient
while nature cures the disease.*

Voltaire

Jeff Bradley is not the kind of person who runs to the doctor
every time he feels some little ache or pain. Quite the con-
trary. But his knees were just killing him. They were stiff,
they ached, and they made strange crackling noises. Finally,
he made an appointment to see the doctor.

When the day of the scheduled visit rolled around, Jeff
was both nervous and a little angry. He didn't like to be sick,
and he liked admitting it even less. He put aside his feelings
of pride, however, because he really needed help. The doctor
would figure out what was wrong and give him medicine to
fix it.

On the examining table, Jeff was asked to bend his knees
this way and that, while the doctor probed his fingers deeply
into the joint. He looked at Jeff with a wry smile. "Well, fella,
looks like old age is creeping up on you. Seems to be arthritis."

After a discussion of what Jeff could expect in the future, Jeff waited for the prescription that would begin to set
things right. Finally he asked, "What's the medicine for this
problem?"

And the doctor told him to take aspirin.

Jeff was angry again. A $30 office visit, his knees still hurting, and the doctor tells him to take *aspirin*. "Some joke," Jeff thought sourly as he drove home.

Well, aspirin *is* ordinary. What Jeff didn't realize is that aspirin is, in fact, the preferred treatment for most kinds of arthritis. In cases of osteoarthritis, it kills pain. But in exactly the right dose, it also can reduce the inflammation that makes rheumatoid arthritis (RA) such a crippler. Taken at regular intervals during the day, it enters the bloodstream and flows through the body, reducing swelling in joints and cooling the inflamed tissue. People with RA often take 10, 12, even 15 tablets a day. At these high doses, it should be taken under a doctor's supervision because it can hit you with some pretty severe side effects.

What Is Aspirin?

This staple of the medicine cabinet came into use as a folk remedy. It first entered medical literature in England in the mid-1700s, when it was reported that the bark of the willow tree cured the "agues"—or fever. The active ingredient in willow bark is a bitter element called salicin. And, in fact, the official name for aspirin is acetylsalicylic acid. Despite its rather humble origin, aspirin is quite a versatile drug; it lessens pain, and reduces both inflammation and fever. These very properties make it the drug of first choice for the treatment of RA.

In a letter to the doctors' magazine *Annals of Internal Medicine,* Joseph Lee Hollander, M.D.—the doctor who quite literally "wrote the book" on arthritis—said: ". . . the term wonder drug now means that we *wonder* if the new drug will ever be as effective as aspirin, and we *wonder* what side effects it will produce. . . . Of the 88 drugs used to treat rheumatoid arthritis 40 or 50 years ago (the early years of rheumatology), few have survived the critical test of use through time. Aspirin, and other salicylates, gold-salt injections, and very few others still have a place."

Although aspirin has been used for about 100 years, it wasn't until 1971 that someone figured out how it works. A British physician discovered that this modest drug can stifle the production of a substance the body manufactures by itself. The substance is a group of fatty acids called prostaglandins. Similar to hormones, they are produced throughout the body and are always released when cells have been damaged. In fact, they have been found in the thick liquid that seeps from inflamed tissues. As far as scientists can tell, our cells don't store prostaglandins but make them right on the spot. Aspirin (and other similar drugs we'll discuss very soon) keeps the prostaglandins from forming, and therefore reduces the impact of the inflammation. Interestingly, if you could inject prostaglandins under someone's skin, they'd develop something just like an inflammation.

You don't need those very large doses of aspirin to stop the formation of prostaglandins. For a brief episode of inflammation—a headache, or sunburn, or whatever—one to two standard-size five-grain tablets will do the trick. The reason those with RA take so many tablets is to keep a fairly constant level of aspirin in the blood to counter their ongoing inflammation.

NOT WITHOUT PROBLEMS

As good as plain old aspirin seems to be, it is not without problems. Some say that if this drug were to be introduced on the market today, the Food and Drug Administration (FDA) would require a prescription for it because of its potentially serious side effects. The most common of these is gastrointestinal problems. Among them are sour stomach, nausea, vomiting, and even ulcers. Damage to the lining of the stomach and/or small intestine usually happens when a person is taking aspirin regularly (four or more days a week) or in large doses (more than 15 tablets a week). A damaged lining then can lead to intestinal bleeding or an ulcer. The reason the stomach and intestine are so vulnerable to damage is that aspirin, while it is inhibiting the production of prostaglandins that make inflammation so painful, also inhibits the prostaglandins that protect the stomach lining.

If you watch television at all, you're probably thinking that these problems could be averted by taking a buffered aspirin. That's what the commercials say. But that's not what at least one doctor has found to be true. Frank L. Lanza,

M.D., tested plain aspirin, buffered aspirin, some prescription drugs, and a specially coated aspirin on 20 healthy volunteers. They took the drugs at their highest recommended doses. What happened? The group taking the buffered aspirin had just as much damage as those who took the plain. The only volunteers who did well were those who took coated aspirin that doesn't dissolve until it gets past your stomach. (By the way, if you drink alcohol while you take aspirin you give your stomach the double whammy because alcohol increases the ulcer-causing potential of aspirin.)

How about Tylenol then? Technically known as acetaminophen, this drug does lessen pain. Therefore, it can be helpful in cases of osteoarthritis. But Tylenol does not have the ability to reduce inflammation, and so doesn't really have a role in the treatment of RA or other types where inflammation is a problem.

In addition to the gastrointestinal side effects, doctors thought for a while that long-term or high-dose use of aspirin caused the kidneys to shrink or could lead to urinary tract infections. However, this speculation hasn't really held up to close scrutiny. A study at the Massachusetts General Hospital Arthritis Clinic looked at people with RA who had been taking aspirin for ten or more years. They found no kidney problems.

But two common side effects that do occur often are ringing in the ears and hearing loss. These seem to develop because of pressure in the inner ear. There is a close relationship between the amount of aspirin you take and the amount of hearing you lose. More aspirin—more loss. However, the problem goes away completely within two or three days of keeping off the drug.

But that's not all, folks. Aspirin and similar anti-inflammatory drugs also wreak havoc with your nutrition. Even in small doses, it can cause you to excrete three times as much vitamin C in your urine as you normally would. And routine use can lead to a folate deficiency. Folate is one of the B-complex vitamins. Concentrated in the spinal fluid, it's a must for calm nerves and clear thinking. In a study of 51 patients with RA, 71 percent had low levels of folate in their blood. All 71 percent were taking aspirin. Moreover, if you develop problems with the lining of your stomach and intestines, you will lose some blood, which will cause you to also lose iron.

This deceptively simple medicine has even *more* side effects. It also can prevent blood from clotting. Worse, it prevents the body from fighting off colds, viruses, and maybe even cancer, by blocking the effect of interferon, another substance produced in our bodies. Scientists at Duke University and Burroughs-Wellcome Research Laboratories, experimenting with the cells of mice, revealed that interferon could not do its work of fighting viruses when aspirin was present. These scientists worry that taking aspirin for a cold may allow the number of cold viruses to multiply more rapidly. They worry that those taking aspirin may be more vulnerable to an entire host of virus-caused diseases. The implications of interferon blockage are enormous for those who take aspirin every day.

New Arthritis Drugs

If aspirin is so dangerous, what can you do to relieve your pain? Some doctors suggest that you switch to one of the aspirinlike drugs that have been flooding the market in recent years. These new drugs—called non-steroidal anti-inflammatory agents—are aspirin's kissin' cousins, acting the same way in the body. They're mild painkillers that fight inflammation.

According to Steve Pickert, M.D., a Maryland family physician, "The proof of these drugs is whether they're more worthwhile than aspirin. Motrin, for example, is easier on the stomach. In fact, it's the drug of first choice in England. In this country, the first-line drug is still aspirin.

"You have to weigh the risk of using these drugs against the benefits. For example, if someone came to me because his shoulder has been hurting for a couple of days, I wouldn't prescribe one of these newer drugs for him. But if he has joint problems so severe he can no longer work, then the benefits of this drug most likely outweigh the risks of taking it," he said.

It seems that as each of these drugs made its debut, some newspaper or magazine ballyhooed it as a new miracle cure for arthritis. The granddaddy of this group is Indocin (indomethacin), which was introduced in 1963. Doctors generally agree that it's not any more effective than aspirin. It does, however, have more serious side effects. In fact, 35 to 50 percent of the people who take this drug develop very bizarre symptoms such as total loss of appetite, nausea, abdominal pain, and painful ulceration of the entire upper gastrointestinal (GI) tract (which sometimes perforates, leading to hemorrhage that can result in anemia). As if these were not enough, other side effects include diarrhea, ulcers in the bowel, hepatitis, jaundice, and severe bone marrow depression. Medical literature suggests in an amazingly understated manner that it is "not a drug to be used routinely."

FIVE MOST OFTEN PRESCRIBED

The next decade, however, brought along a milder group of aspirinlike drugs that includes Motrin (ibuprofen), Naprosyn (naproxen), Clinoril (sulindac), Nalfon (fenoprofen), and Tolectin (tolmetin). All non-steroidal anti-inflammatory agents, they are almost identical quintuplets in the family of arthritis drugs. They're all taken orally and absorbed directly into the bloodstream in about an hour. They travel throughout the body and have been found in synovial tissue, spinal fluid, and saliva. Usually, they're prescribed for RA, osteoarthritis, and ankylosing spondylitis. Even though they work the same way, they're chemically different. For that reason, some people react better to one than to the others. Usually you'll know after taking a drug for a week whether it's going to harm your gastrointestinal tract or not.

Let's make a quick rundown of each to note how each works and what any possible side effects might be.

Motrin (ibuprofen) was introduced first in Great Britain in the late 1960s and in the United States in 1974. It is a weak but effective anti-inflammatory. Once in the system, it passes slowly into the synovial area, where it remains long after the amount in the bloodstream has diminished. Even though its side effects are supposed to be less than those of aspirin, 15 percent of those taking the drug nevertheless develop symptoms severe enough to cause them to discontinue it.

One unexpected side effect of Motrin (and a chemically

identical drug, Brufen, available only in Great Britain) is that it can cause your hair to fall out. In a letter to the editor in the *Journal of the American Medical Association*, a doctor reported that of 21 patients who were taking Motrin, 15 had reported hair thinning or loss. "It seems that ibuprofen may affect the protein (in the hair) in a manner that causes fragility or brittleness when the hair is exposed to straighteners, processes, or permanent wave procedures. This brittleness causes the hair to break off at the epidermal (skin) level and does not affect the hair root." His patients were switched to another one of the quintuplet drugs, and their hair began growing again.

Naprosyn (naproxen) is easier to live with than aspirin because you have to take it only twice a day. It is often prescribed for RA and seems especially beneficial for ankylosing spondylitis. Generally, it's the drug in this group that gives people the least trouble with side effects.

Clinoril (sulindac) is prescribed for all the major kinds of arthritis, including gout and painful shoulder. It's a mild painkiller and works mostly because it reduces inflammation. It's been found to be as effective as aspirin for the treatment of osteoarthritis. Unfortunately, side effects include diarrhea or constipation, abdominal pain, nausea and, less frequently, ulceration and consequent blood loss.

Nalfon (fenoprofen) is similar to those drugs just described. Side effects to look for include: indigestion, constipation, nausea, vomiting, heartburn, itching, skin rash, fluid retention, ringing in the ears, blurred vision.

Tolectin (tolmetin) is approved for the treatment of rheumatoid and juvenile rheumatoid arthritis, and osteoarthritis. It is considered as effective as aspirin, but with fewer side effects. Nevertheless, 25 to 40 percent of those taking the drug do report having undesirable symptoms, with 5 to 10 percent made so uncomfortable they must discontinue using it.

BUTE THE BRUTE

Bute stands for Butazolidin (phenylbutazone). It's a beaut all right. This drug has been around the track since 1949—the racetrack, that is, where it's been used on horses. But it's not a winner.

On page 1000 of the *Physician's Drug Manual,* a book that's in almost every doctor's office, you'll find this description of Butazolidin and Butazolidin Alka:

> *Initiating therapy—Use only in patients unresponsive to other therapies . . . warn patients not to exceed dosage and to immediately report sore throat, skin rashes, dyspepsia, epigastric pain, unusual bleeding, black or tarry stools, weight gain, or edema.*

And under "Warnings and Precautions," you'll find the following:

> *Drug toxicity—Severe or fatal reactions may occur especially in patients over 40 years of age; elderly are at greatest risk.*

> *Upper GI tests—Should be performed in patients with persistent or severe dyspepsia: peptic ulcer, bleeding, and perforation may occur.*

> *Systemic lupus erythematosus—Discontinue drug if symptoms are activated.*

> *Leukemia—Causal relationship has not been firmly established, but cases have been reported.*

Perforated ulcers? Leukemia? Here's a case where the treatment is surely worse than the disease. And, in the words of Al Jolson, "You ain't seen nothin' yet." Butazolidin can cause the bone marrow to go so haywire that no blood cells develop, resulting in aplastic anemia. Because the condition can be fatal, the person taking the drug requires frequent blood tests. The drug has also been known to cause jaundice, blurred vision, and asthma attacks. Side effects develop in as many as 45 percent of the people taking this drug.

For all of this trouble, the drug is *less* effective than aspirin for treating arthritis.

Butazolidin should be avoided like the plague—as should a drug closely related to it: Tandearil (oxyphen-butazone).

More New Entries

Thus we see that the majority of the drugs used to treat arthritis are either aspirin or similar to it—mild painkillers that work against inflammation, but often result in gastrointestinal problems.

But, like the guy who builds a better mousetrap, there is a medical researcher who is creating a better aspirin. One without the side effects. John R.J. Sorenson, Ph.D., working at the University of Arkansas Medical School in Little Rock, has suggested that if you combine aspirin with copper you'd get such a drug. His studies have shown that aspirin has a chemical reaction which causes it to bind with a metal that is naturally present in our bodies. This process, called chelation, allows a chemical (such as aspirin) to latch on to a metal (such as copper) and carry it away.

Dr. Sorenson thinks that when aspirin removes copper from the stomach lining, trouble begins. It is the lack of copper that allows the tissue to become damaged and ulcers to form. It seems the addition of copper to aspirin eliminates the problem. He also believes that copper may be the clue to what makes aspirin effective in arthritis treatment. "Evidence exists that copper turns off pro-inflammation prostaglandins while turning on the synthesis of anti-inflammation prostaglandins," he explains.

Dr. Sorenson says the combination of aspirin and copper is the real medicine that repairs damaged tissue and reduces inflammation, rather than aspirin alone. Copper does not reduce the synthesis of prostaglandins, but rather changes the kinds of prostaglandins that are made. In one test, the copper-aspirin combo was 20 times more effective than just aspirin.

It may be some time before you can easily find copper aspirinate (which is not a prescription drug) on the shelves of your local drugstore. Dr. Sorenson is currently putting the experimental drug through the many tests required by the FDA. However, you can supplement your diet with 2 milligrams of copper (the Recommended Dietary Allowance) and watch for signs of improvement.

Two additional new entries in the field of arthritis drugs have just been approved at this writing. One, called Oraflex (benoxaprofen), is a non-steroidal anti-inflammatory that differs from the others in that it not only reduces inflammation but also may slow the disease process itself.

You may remember in the discussion of RA that the cartilage, and even bone, in a joint can be destroyed by enzymes released by the cells of our own immune system. These cells misread those tissues as dangerous foreign substances, and rush to the joint to attack them. Oraflex is supposed to stop these cells before they get to the joint. It also acts to slow the production of prostaglandins, but is not as strong as aspirin in doing so.

Like other drugs in this category, Oraflex also can cause gastrointestinal problems, including ulcers and bleeding. In addition, if you take the drug and go out in the sunshine, your skin can burn or itch, and your nails can fall out.

The other new drug is Feldene (piroxicam). It, too, slows the production of prostaglandins and halts the migration of white blood cells to inflamed joints. What's different about this drug is that it belongs to an entirely new family of drugs called "oxicams," while all the other aspirinlike drugs are in the chemical family called carboxylic acids. It's said to be less irritating than aspirin, but 20 percent of the people taking it develop gastrointestinal problems anyway. About 5 percent are forced to discontinue using it.

Like so many of the drugs introduced in the last few years, Oraflex and Feldene come highly touted.

At this writing, reports of serious side effects of both drugs are surfacing, and a number of deaths have been reported. Extreme caution is the watchword with these two new drugs.

What to Do

If you are taking aspirin or any of the more expensive aspirinlike drugs, do pay special attention to any signs of stomach disorder. If you *must* take these drugs, ask your doctor to recommend the lowest possible dosage. Take them with meals or with a glass of milk. And be sure to supplement your diet with plenty of vitamin C, which you excrete at abnormally high rates when taking aspirin and the like. If you have had any gastric bleeding in the past, also supplement your diet with iron.

An additional word of warning: The new group of anti-inflammatory drugs were developed as an alternative to the high doses of aspirin required to treat RA, doses which almost always end up causing a shredded stomach lining. However, doctors seem to have fallen head over heels for them. Instead of limiting them strictly to the treatment of RA, many doctors prescribe them willy-nilly for any little ache or pain. If you do not have RA, you do not need these expensive drugs. Instead, try baggie therapy, rest, exercise, or a good book to divert your mind. Go on a diet to lighten the load on the joint that's bothering you. Supplement your diet with bone meal and vitamin D. If you're feeling desperate, take an occasional aspirin. But don't fall into the trap of taking a drug that's too big for your disease. It's like burning down the house to barbecue the spareribs.

Steroids: The Quick Fix

Cortisone was discovered and introduced into medical treatment in the 1950s. It was hailed as a miracle drug—indeed, it seemed to be too good to be true. And it was.

Cortisone is a hormone produced in our own bodies by the adrenals, two little glands that sit—one each—atop the kidneys. Scientists isolated cortisone from the other secretions produced by the glands, and learned to synthesize it in a laboratory. When people with RA were first given this drug, their symptoms disappeared, literally, almost overnight. Folks who had spent years confined to a chair or bed were

A SAFE NEW DRUG—MAYBE

If you must take strong arthritis drugs, then so be it. But it seems there may be an alternative just over the horizon. Called Orgotein, it's made from a substance found in all mammalian cells. So far, it's been approved for use only on animals.

A study published in the British medical journal, the *Lancet,* reports that 30 people with active rheumatoid arthritis showed improvement after 12 weeks of Orgotein injections. The scientists conducting the study concluded that the drug was at least superior to aspirin and, unlike cortisone, it seemed safe.

Mark Saiffer, M.D., who is helping to develop the drug in the United States, says that the drug is a powerful anti-inflammatory that can produce a six-month remission after a full course of treatment. It is usually injected directly into the joint. The drug, made from beef liver, is "nontoxic, does not cause problems in the gastrointestinal tract or with the blood, but may present some unwanted side effects in people who have certain allergies," he explains.

The drug is being studied for future testing by the Food and Drug Administration.

suddenly up and about. Their limbs moved and their spirits soared.

Unfortunately, in the next few years, the drug showed itself to be just as dangerous as it was wonderful. Doctors discovered that their patients who took large amounts, especially for a long time, developed some very serious side effects that never were anticipated. These include stomach ulcers, loss of muscle tone, "moon faces," a so-called "buffalo hump" of fat at the upper back, hair growth on the faces of women, osteoporosis, inability of wounds to heal, cataracts, high blood pressure, greater appetite, emotional depression, even psychosis. Oh boy.

The drugs that produce this wonderful relief from inflammation and the correspondingly terrible side effects are Aristocort, Decadron, Delta-cortef, Hydrocortone, and Metacorten.

Chances are, you're not taking a steroid drug unless you have a pretty bad case of RA. However, some doctors do tend to overprescribe, so ask whether it's possible for you to switch to something milder, or to reduce your dosage. Even if the answer is yes, you won't be able to stop taking the drug immediately. You see, after taking steroids for a time, your own adrenal glands just shut down. After all, you're supplying the hormone, so they don't have to. At any rate, if you were to just stop suddenly, your body wouldn't be able to pick up the slack. Therefore, doctors generally have you reduce the dose, then space out how often you take the drug—for example, taking it every day, then every other day, then twice a week, and then not at all.

By the way, random injections of cortisone directly into a painful joint do not produce these dreadful side effects. Often a painful case of bursitis or a joint really hot with osteoarthritis will respond dramatically with one injection. The inflammation is suppressed and the cycle of pain is broken. Because of its very brief stay in the body, the drug doesn't have a chance to do a lot of damage. Keep in mind, however, that applying ice often produces the same relief.

If you're stuck taking steroids, there are still things you can do to help reduce the severity of the side effects.

Swelling can be reduced by eliminating salt from your diet. Taking a potassium supplement may also help.

Muscle wasting can be reduced through exercise.

Osteoporosis, a condition where the bone thins and becomes so brittle it easily breaks, also can be held in check by supplementing the diet with additional calcium and vitamin D.

Slow-healing wounds are effectively treated by taking vitamin A supplements and by spreading vitamin A ointment gently over the sore. A report in the *Annals of Surgery* tells of an 18-year-old girl with lupus who developed an ulcer on her leg after bumping it. It remained unhealed for some time. However, new tissue began to form in only three days after applying vitamin A ointment three times a day.

Depression has been found to respond to very high doses of vitamin C, according to several doctors writing in *Pediatrics* magazine. Working in Florence, Italy, they reported they were able to reverse the severe depression of a five-year-old who was taking steroids by giving her vitamin C intravenously.

Surprisingly, steroids are not the heaviest drug artillery used against arthritis. In fact, compared to the next level of drugs, they're just a paltry potshot.

There's Gold in Them Thar Pills

One of the latest developments on the drug scene is a medication called Ridaura, a pill containing gold. It's considered a big deal by doctors because, until the development of this pill, gold always had to be given via injection. (And it's considered a big deal by Wall Street prognosticators, who predict that world-wide sales may reach $1 billion.) The pills, taken daily for treatment of RA, are supposed to have fewer side effects than injections because they are less powerful.

Gold—either taken orally or by injection—is considered a "remission-inducing drug," which means it has an effect that is sustained even after you stop taking it. It can suppress or possibly prevent the symptoms of arthritis, but it cannot cure the disease.

One can't help but wonder how gold came to be used as a drug. What mad scientist came up with the nutty idea of shooting gold into someone's body? Rumor has it that it was first recommended by Abu Moussa the Wise back in the eighth century. Some 1,100 years later, a scientist named Robert Koch showed that gold cyanide prevented tuberculosis (TB) germs from growing. Probably thinking that the inflammation of RA was similar to TB, several scientists in Germany and France experimented with the effects of gold salts on arthritis. And, quite remarkably, it worked. But to this day, no one can explain why.

Unlike steroids or aspirin, the beneficial effect of gold doesn't appear for weeks or even months. When given by injection, the dose is increased gradually each week, until a maximum of 50 milligrams is reached. The injections are painful and can have serious side effects. The most common of these are sores in the mouth or on other mucous membranes, and skin rashes. But sometimes extremely serious side effects develop—problems of the blood that can result in aplastic anemia or leave you wide open to infection. Kidneys can become damaged, causing you to excrete abnormally large amounts of protein. Because of these dangers, people taking gold must have frequent blood tests and urinalysis.

One-quarter to one-half of all people on gold therapy develop some side effects. In fact, it's believed that you have to reach the point of toxicity before a remission can occur. Nevertheless, about 75 percent who take the drug feel better for it. X rays show that joint damage is slowed or even stopped, and that gold may prevent damage in joints that probably would have become involved. People taking it have a stronger grip and less morning stiffness—two criteria for measuring improvement.

Penicillamine and Chloroquine

A second remission-inducing drug is penicillamine. Although its name leads you to believe that it's an antibiotic like penicillin, it is not. It is, however, made from the urine of people taking penicillin. Again, nobody understands why the drug works. What scientists do know is that it latches on to heavy metals and causes the body to excrete them. Like gold, it requires several months to work. The side effects of penicillamine are gruesome. They include explosive vomiting, a loss of taste, sores on mucous membranes, excretion of protein in urine, bone marrow problems, gastrointestinal grief, skin rashes, and some that are even more serious—such as lupus and myasthenia gravis.

The third in the triad of remission-inducing medications is chloroquine, which is actually a drug used to treat malaria. It is marketed under the names Aralen, Avloclor, and Resochin. A similar drug, hydroxychloroquine, is sold as Plaquenil. Taken orally, they require anywhere from three to six months to work.

Generally, they are used to treat chronic, active RA. Taken over a long period of time, they can create some unwanted symptoms. These include skin rashes and sores, hair loss, and the tendency for the skin to burn badly if you go out into the sunlight. All these problems disappear when you stop taking the drug. But one side effect—the most serious—does not go away. The chloroquines can cause an eye abnormality called retinopathy, which can result in blindness. To head off this problem, people taking these drugs must have their eyes examined anywhere from two to four times a year.

Hormone Therapy

In addition to all these drugs, medical science is also experimenting with sex hormones. Doctors have known for a long time that if a woman with RA became pregnant, her symptoms would just about disappear. She'd enter a remission that lasted as long as the pregnancy.

Presumably, then, if you gave women with RA the same amount of hormones that develop naturally during pregnancy, their arthritis might go away, too. And that is exactly the experiment tried by Harold Varon, M.D., at the Baylor University Medical Center in Dallas, Texas. Working with 14 women who had active RA for as long as 6 to 23 years, Dr. Varon gave them weekly injections of estrogen and progesterone. They improved quite dramatically, with swelling and pain diminishing, and range of motion improving. X rays also showed that there was a rapid reduction in osteoporosis, and that joint displacement (subluxation) also improved. None of the women experienced a flare-up while on the hormones.

And while the results may be quite exciting, we should all remember that this treatment is basically a steroid therapy, a therapy that seems to have inevitable drawbacks in the long run.

*   *   *

The Arthritis Foundation estimates that people spend $1.3 *billion* a year seeking relief from arthritis with drugs. Most only relieve the symptoms and do nothing to halt the disease. Many have side effects so severe they threaten life. Until the cause of this disease is nailed down, there probably can be no cure, unless someone accidentally stumbles upon one. (Soon, we hope!)

Therefore, the wise person will always try to trade down on medicine, substituting ever milder drugs until you reach the point where you take none at all. For some, this strategy is not feasible. If you have a very severe form of arthritis, instead work to strengthen your body with an excellent diet, rest, and careful exercise. And remember, the proper vitamin and mineral supplements can counter the side effects of aspirin and steroids to a great degree. Keep trying and keep working. It will pay off.

16

THE OPTION OF SURGERY

"The doctor showed me two X rays—before and after—taken of someone with a condition similar to mine. Then he explained what the operation would be like, how much pain I could expect, what kinds of anesthetic are available, and how long it would take me to get back on my feet. I asked a lot of questions and he gave me straight answers," explains Linda Halkins, an attractive young artist recovering from surgery on her foot.

The decision to undergo arthritis surgery can be difficult because it is elective surgery. Nobody is going to drag you into the operating room muttering about matters of life and death. You have to decide you want this surgery, and the option can seem very frightening. Linda decided in favor of surgery because her condition—a splayed joint at the ball of her foot—was getting to be a problem. "I realized I could never tour England on vacation because it means a lot of walking. There were lots of little things, too. I'd put off seeing other people involved in my work if it meant walking to another office. Finally I figured I'd trade four to six weeks of recuperation for getting my freedom back.

"I was nervous about the operation, but it wasn't really that bad. After the doctor stitched up my foot—but before it began to swell—he asked me to look at it. It was *beautiful*. It looked just like a regular foot! Now I'm waiting for the bandages to come off so I can go out and buy a new pair of shoes. Pretty ones!" beams Linda.

Plastic Joints and Band-Aids

The range of arthritis surgery is very large, including everything from Linda's fairly common ostectomy to the latest "band-aid" knee surgery and on to total hip replacement. Until recently, surgery was not performed unless all other treatments had failed. Today, however, new surgical techniques allow for the early removal of chronically inflamed tissue before any permanent damage is done, as well as for reconstruction or replacement of joints that have been destroyed by arthritis.

Not everyone who wants arthritis surgery, however, can have it. Several factors can prohibit it, including infections, overweight, serious heart disease, diabetes, and emphysema. Also, if someone with rheumatoid arthritis (RA) is having a serious flare-up, surgery is usually postponed until the episode subsides.

Age, however, is not a deterrent to arthritis surgery. Healthy people in their 80s and even 90s can tolerate anesthesia as well as younger folks, according to Jovan L. Djokovic, M.D., and John Hedley-Whyte, M.D., as reported in the *Journal of the American Medical Association*. And that's good news, since it's usually the older person who suffers most from the accumulated effects of the disease.

Let's take a look at some of the more common procedures available today.

Synovectomy is the removal of the synovial membrane. After chronic inflammation, this membrane can become thick and shaggy, filling the entire joint space and eventually destroying the joint. Often, it is removed by opening the entire joint, then cutting out the membrane. Today, however, a procedure called *arthroscopy* has become a more popular, more comfortable, and more economical alternative.

With arthroscopy (the band-aid surgery), a tiny fiber-optic viewing instrument can be inserted right into the joint. Some doctors attach a tiny television camera to it. Other instruments are then inserted through additional very small holes to carry out the actual tissue removal. After traditional surgery, you could expect to have a scar anywhere from three to six inches long, a stay of several days in the hospital, plus several weeks of rehabilitation. After arthroscopy, however, you usually can leave the hospital in a couple of hours, walk in 24 hours, and be back to normal activity in weeks. The surgery is a bit more expensive than the old method, but you do eliminate the cost of a hospital stay, and can resume work sooner. This surgery is available for knees, wrists, and elbows.

Some doctors think that arthroscopy is the first-choice treatment for people who have persistent knee synovitis. Others, however, warn that the tissue can grow back and become inflamed again.

In addition to arthroscopy, surgeons can perform a variety of other treatments including:

Mold arthroplasty, which involves opening the joint, scraping clean the bones that meet in the joint, and capping each with a metal or plastic head. The two caps are then joined by a "spacer" that acts as a hinge.

Joint fusion (arthrodesis) freezes the bones together, effectively removing the joint. It substitutes balance and stability for flexibility.

Joint replacement means exactly what it says. Artificial joints are available for the hips, wrists, elbows, shoulders, knees, and fingers. In the United States alone, 100,000 hips and 50,000 knees are replaced in a year's time. Most people who get new joints are usually thrilled with the results. They feel less pain and get around much better than before. However, there are some problems. Loosening of the replacement happens to about one in four. Improved bone cement may rectify this problem in the future. Moreover, those who have hip joint or knee surgery are more likely to develop phlebitis than the general public.

Natural Boosters for Faster Healing

If you choose to undergo surgery for arthritis, there are a number of ways you can help yourself recover quickly and without incident. First, as always, is nutrition. Hard as it may be to believe, your nutritional requirements are actually greater when you're lying in a hospital bed than when you're going about your normal daily activities.

As soon as you have decided on surgery, start building up your body so it will have the nutritional reserves it needs. Begin by supplementing your diet with a multiple vitamin/mineral supplement of at least the Recommended Dietary Allowance (RDA) level. And don't expect your doctor to tell you if your nutritional status is up to snuff. Erroneous assumptions about the nutritional status of patients contribute to the epidemic of physician-induced malnutrition in hospital patients. Basing his conclusions on broad hospital experience, Charles E. Butterworth, Jr., M.D., director of the nutrition program at the University of Alabama and former chairman of the Council of Foods and Nutrition of the American Medical Association, wrote in *Nutrition Today* magazine, "I suspect, as a matter of fact, that one of the largest pockets of unrecognized malnutrition in America . . . exists not in rural slums or urban ghettos, but in the private rooms and wards of the big city hospitals. . . . I am convinced that iatrogenic (physician-caused) malnutrition has become a significant factor in determining the outcome of illness for many patients."

One doctor who does size up the nutritional status of his future surgery patients is August Daro, M.D., of Chicago, Illinois. "Foremost is the importance of sound diet. Eating the wrong foods will give you far too many calories and not enough protein, which heads you straight for the protein malnutrition that is so common in hospital patients. Be sure to eat enough protein," Dr. Daro warns. Just remember to go with low-fat foods like skim milk, fish, and poultry rather than the standard steak, chops, and hamburger route.

Once you've completed surgery, you will be burning more calories than ever because your metabolism will be set at full throttle. All the energy you require can come from only two sources—the food you eat and the carbohydrates, fat, and protein stored in your body.

The body first uses up the available carbohydrates for energy. Within 8 to 16 hours after eating your last meal (probably six in the evening before surgery), total carbohydrate stores will be completely exhausted. As you can see, trouble can begin quite early. Your body also needs protein, important not only for day-to-day survival but vital for emergency tissue repair. Moreover, it cannot be manufactured from either stored carbohydrates or fats. If dietary intake is inadequate to meet the increased repair needs after surgery, the body steals protein from muscles.

Most healthy men need about 55 grams of protein (the equivalent of six ounces of lean chicken) daily for normal body function. Healthy women need 45 grams. Postsurgical patients need much, much more for urgent tissue repair—at least 100 grams a day or more, depending on the extent of the operation.

For each gram of protein to be properly utilized by the body, it must be accompanied by 25 calories from fats and/or carbohydrates. This combined nutrition results in a need for about 3,000 calories a day, minimum.

Sure, you could just eat more while you're in the hospital. But chances are, you won't. Presurgery jitters, poor appetite after surgery, hospital food that's unappealing, prescribed drugs, missed meals, the tea-toast-gelatin routine, or being forbidden to eat because of lab tests all conspire to keep you underfed and undernourished.

With a low intake of protein and calories—not to mention missing vitamins and minerals—the body simply can't make the necessary repairs. For that reason, no matter how little hunger you feel, do attempt to eat as much of the food put before you as possible. If you can manage to get permission from your doctor, snack on high-protein foods like yogurt or whole-grain cereals.

VITAMIN C

The soaring needs for protein and calories are accompanied by the need for additional vitamins and minerals. Vitamin C (ascorbic acid) is the chief healing vitamin because it is essential for the manufacture of collagen, a tough, fibrous substance which gives strength to new tissue by cementing cells together, making healing possible, and preventing the layers of the wound from splitting apart. Vitamin C also heals wounds indirectly by encouraging the tiny blood vessels called capillaries to renew themselves in the wound area, bringing with them red blood cells, nutrients, and anti-bodies that fight infectious bacteria.

Large amounts of vitamin C are normally stored in the adrenal cortex and promote overall recovery by helping that gland to produce certain hormones which protect the entire body against all kinds of stress, including surgery. However, these stores are rapidly depleted not only by the increased stress of surgery but also by any disease, fever, or infection that may accompany it. In fact, the more severe the stress, the faster the rate of vitamin C depletion. If your stores are inadequate, your recovery could be prolonged a week or more.

The *minimum required dose of vitamin C for wound-healing is 500 milligrams a day,* compared to the RDA of 60 milligrams for a healthy person. Needs may go up to 3 grams (3,000 milligrams) a day or higher during the initial stages of healing. Because vitamin C is water soluble and the excess beyond tissue saturation is passed out in the urine, doses should be given at several intervals throughout the day, rather than all of it taken in one huge swallow.

VITAMIN A

Just as vitamin C sparks collagen formation, vitamin A influences the rate at which the collagen is laid down between cells, and so it, too, encourages the growth and repair of tissue. Vitamin A's larger role is to maintain the health of the epithelium, tissues that line organs and cover the body. When those tissues are wounded—as in surgery—epithelial cells at the edge of the wound begin to migrate over it, leapfrogging to bridge the gap. Moreover, it's been shown that vitamin A in large doses helps strengthen the body's immune response. After surgery, your own immune system often goes into a slump, leaving you dangerously open to infection. However, vitamin A can block that depression and act as an immuno-*stimulant,* according to a study performed by doctors at the University of Oxford in Great Britain.

The body manufactures vitamin A from carotene in green, leafy vegetables and from deep yellow vegetables such as squash, carrots, and sweet potatoes. It's also found in beef liver, cheese, eggs, and milk. *Doses of 10,000 International*

*Units (I.U.) of vitamin A a day meet the approximate needs
of someone who has just undergone surgery,* as compared to
4,000 or 5,000 in the general population.

B VITAMINS

The need for B vitamins also increases after surgery.
Although this group of vitamins always go hand in hand, each
specific vitamin plays a specific role in healing after surgery.

Both **folate** and **vitamin B$_{12}$** help maintain the red blood
cells—an important job because these deliver vital nutrients
to all cells, including those involved in wound-healing. Either
because the body needs much more of the nutrients or because the patient is eating much less, deficiencies of these
two vitamins are most likely to crop up in hospital popula-
tions. So pay special attention to your need for folate and
B$_{12}$. *The recommended therapeutic dose for folate is 1 milli-
gram; for vitamin B$_{12}$ it's 4 micrograms.*

Thiamine, along with folate, liberates energy from the
carbohydrates you eat and those stored in your body. The
more carbohydrates in your diet (and that's what is in your
intravenous tube), the more thiamine you need. *The recommended therapeutic dose is 10 milligrams.*

Both **pyridoxine** and **pantothenate** appear to play an important role in the formation of antibodies, which help guard
you against infection. *The recommended therapeutic dose for
pyridoxine is 2 to 25 milligrams. The recommended
therapeutic dose for pantothenate is 20 milligrams.*

Riboflavin and **niacin** are both powerful friends—with
one helping your body to get the most from protein and the
other working to release the goodness of both protein and
carbohydrates. *The recommended therapeutic dose for
riboflavin is 5 to 10 milligrams. The recommended
therapeutic dose for niacin is 100 milligrams.*

ZINC AND COPPER

Minerals, too, are basic to the healing process, and one
of the most important is zinc. One study found that surgical
patients given zinc supplements had healthier-looking new
tissue in their rapidly healing wounds. It's not too surprising

that a deficiency of zinc can lead to slower healing and, therefore, greater possibility of wound infection. The standard RDA for zinc is 15 milligrams, but *for therapeutic purposes increase daily supplementation to 30 milligrams.*

When zinc deficiency does occur, it is quite likely to go hand in hand with a deficit of copper, also essential to health. Copper is needed to forge myelin, the protective sheath that surrounds nerve fibers, and to aid the body in iron absorption.

Textbooks have traditionally stated that the average diet provides more than enough copper to meet the 2 milligrams needed to replace daily losses. But many hospital patients simply don't get enough of either copper or zinc.

A study by Leslie M. Klevay, M.D., and other researchers conducted for the U.S. Department of Agriculture and the University of North Dakota, looked at 20 hospital diets, as well as diets consumed by the general public. The startling results showed that hospital diets averaged 0.76 milligrams of copper a day—that's a full 60 percent below the 2-milligram requirement—and that zinc levels averaged only 9.4 milligrams per day, 35 percent below the 15-milligram requirement.

These researchers are convinced that the average diet—eaten in the hospital or elsewhere—does not provide enough zinc or copper. The therapeutic level of copper has not been established, but be sure you get at least the recommended 2 milligrams per day by eating foods high in copper, such as beef liver, mushrooms, whole wheat, and bananas.

IRON

A poor diet, along with the blood loss of surgery, can also mean that your body does not have enough iron to get along. Iron is important because it delivers vital oxygen throughout the body via red blood cells. *The recommended therapeutic dosage of iron is 10 milligrams for men and 18 milligrams for women.* Good food sources include lean meats, beef liver, beans, legumes, nuts, green leafy vegetables, and whole grains.

Survival Tips for Hospital Food

Hospitals are a very unnatural environment where your emotions seem to swerve from sheer terror to utter boredom, with little rest between. After your operation, when the doctor finally stops by to say that everything is fine and you'll be up and dancing in no time, your emotions generally come to rest at the boredom end of the scale. Magazines. Television. A visitor. And three meals a day. Those meals become more than just sustenance; they become a focal point in the day—things happen before lunch or after dinner. Meals are entertainment, a topic of conversation with your roommate, something to complain about and look forward to.

Despite all of this sudden importance, hospital food is usually no better or worse than that served by the local diner. Wheaties for breakfast, hamburgers for lunch, and stew for dinner. While the familiarity of the menu may be somewhat comforting, the food, itself, may not be nutritious enough to meet your postsurgical requirements.

When the nurses' aide shows up at bedside with the menu for tomorrow, get out your pencil and check off the foods that offer lots of protein, vitamins, and minerals. In addition to your orange juice and Wheaties, check off a soft-boiled egg. Make the toast whole wheat. Skip the coffee and order a glass of milk. Do the same for lunch, keeping your eye out for a side of cottage cheese rather than french fries. Ask for some fruit for dessert.

The big event of the hospital day is usually dinner—often served long before sundown so that you'll be good and hungry by bedtime. It's almost always a traditional meal: meat, potatoes, a vegetable, bread or a dinner roll, and some sort of sweet for dessert. If you can manage it, choose broiled or baked meat over the fried, and light meat (chicken or fish) over red. Scrap the gravy. See if you can get a fresh salad in place of the canned string beans. Order milk with your meal and skip the Jello-O.

In addition to clever ordering, you can supplement the institutional food with assorted goodies from home. Bring along some wheat germ and dried fruit to sprinkle on your oatmeal. Ask your most faithful visitor to smuggle in some yogurt. Keep herb tea bags in your bedside stand so you can have a cup of something hot and soothing while you're watching the afternoon soaps and game shows.

Sure, eating well in the hospital is a little bit of trouble. But, remember, you'll be on your feet a lot faster if you follow this sensible routine.

17

LIVING WELL IS THE BEST REVENGE

Here you are with arthritis, a chronic disease for which no cure has yet been found. But, if you've followed the suggestions in this book, you should be feeling pretty good about yourself and your prospects for the future. You've probably begun experimenting with the various diets offered. With luck, you've already found the perfect one for you. Chances are, your new, custom-made exercise program has already begun to pay off with greater range of motion and less joint stiffness. And maybe you've undertaken some natural pain-relief measures that have allowed you to cut down on those expensive drugs. The program seems complete.

Yet, for many who did not bring arthritis under control before joints became permanently damaged, there's still one more hurdle to vault—coping with daily activities. Climbing stairs, getting out of a deep chair, lifting a heavy pot, scratching your back, bending over to retrieve a dropped coin—the day is filled with quite ordinary tasks to be performed by your no-longer-so-ordinary joints. How, then, do you cope?

As with so many important things in life, the *will* to do something is the primary factor. Take a look at the courage shown by the French painter Pierre Auguste Renoir. His impressionist paintings were full of bright colors dissolving in the sunlight. As objects, he chose parties, dances, happy revelry. Who could know that he suffered with rheumatoid arthritis, or that his hands were almost useless knots of pain? How did he manage to paint at all, no less brilliantly? In his day (he died in 1919), there were no exotic drugs or joint replacements, and pitifully few mechanical aids. And so, he devised his own.

If his arm couldn't move his brush freely over the canvas, he moved the canvas under his brush. Using rollers, he raised and lowered the surface so that he could reach every part. His thumb was virtually useless. How can you hold a paint brush without a thumb? He devised an artificial one out of bandages. And he painted.

Today, thank heavens, there is an army to help us, made up of physical therapists, doctors, manufacturers, and fellow arthritis sufferers who have created tools and techniques to help get us through the day quite independently.

EASY DOES IT

Let's begin with some easy-to-remember techniques that will help you take the strain and pain out of a number of common activities. In the kitchen, for example, remember to pick up a pot with both hands—one holding the handle, the other (protected by an oven mitt) under the pot. You might also consider purchasing two-handled pots. If that seems too much of an expense, try using a deep-fry wire basket in your pot. When the food is cooked, you lift it out in the basket—eliminating the weight of the pot and the water in it. When you later carry that pot full of water to the sink, hold it as close to your body as you can.

Still in the kitchen, try to open jars with the heel of your hand rather than with your fingers. Buy a kitchen stool—the tall kind that will put you at the right height for countertop working. Remember to sit on it when you are chopping, slicing, etc. Also, use it when you do the ironing.

In any work area, organize frequently used objects so they are at chest height. If possible, slide rather than lift them. Even better, drop rather than place them. (Common sense is essential here, of course. This technique works better for sorting laundry than glassware.)

When you're sitting, raise your knees higher than your hips by using a footstool. Driving, remember to sit close to the pedals. Use a wedge-shaped cushion under your thighs to elevate your knees.

When lifting, there are only two hard-and-fast rules. Keep the object close to you and bend your knees. Here's why. If the thing you want to lift weighs 40 pounds and it's placed at your feet, you will be lifting only that 40 pounds. But, move that object three feet away from you and try to lift it from there. You can't. That's because it now weighs the equivalent of 400 pounds. Therefore, always get as close as you can. Keeping your back straight, squat down. Let the thigh muscles do the work—not your spine. If you begin to lose your balance, let the object drop.

Lots of tools are available, too, to make tasks easier and less painful. Dressing and undressing, for example, is infinitely easier if you replace the buttons and zippers on your garments with Velcro strips. You can also use dressing sticks, which are shaped something like a wooden coat hanger, with a rubber stopper at one end. They help position sleeves for you, so you get your arms into them easily. And don't forget to try a long-handled shoehorn, or even elastic shoelaces.

For grooming, there are long-handled combs that allow you to comb your hair with your arm no higher than chest level. Long-handled toothbrushes can be purchased, too. And washing is easier for some when they use a terry cloth mitt that has a pocket for soap. (If you don't drop it, you don't have to pick it up!)

For dining, a fork, spoon, and knife with a built-up handle make "the slips 'tween cup and lip" much fewer. There's also a line of dinnerware designed for those with arthritis in their hands. The cups are double handled. The plates are made with a decided undercut of the inside edge so that you can push food against it, and nab each morsel. For glasses, do consider stemware. You can rest the weight of the liquid in your glass against your entire hand, while the stem slides easily to the center of your palm.

Other handy gadgets include long tongs with magnetic ends, built-up pencils, book stands, raised toilet seats, and grab bars in the tub. Another goodie—one you can make yourself—is a key extension. To make turning the key easier for you, simply screw a block of wood to the end of it. The screw fits where a key ring would normally go.

Think about adapting your furniture, too. If you have trouble sitting and rising, you can raise a chair by placing blocks under the legs. For stability, the blocks should be routed out in the center, so the legs fit snugly inside. There are mechanical chairs, too, that—with the push of a button—push you into a standing position.

Beds should be firm. These, too, can be raised with blocks. And never (not ever!) sleep with a pillow under your flexed knees. You'll just create more problems. If your neck is what's giving you the trouble, there are pillows shaped like a butterfly, allowing softness without forcing your neck up into a painful angle.

*   *   *

Finally (saving the best for last), find yourself a support group. Many Ys have "arthritis swims." Try visiting one. High school night courses offer a way to make new friends while learning a skill that intrigues you. Garden clubs, sewing circles, church groups all meet regularly. Join one and you'll have something to look forward to every week or month. Volunteer your time—reading for the Children's Hour at the local library, or for the blind of the community.

Maybe you can't do everything you once did. And maybe some days you can't do anything. So be it. But there's still a whole world of excitement and fun, satisfaction and hope. And you're part of it.

Appendix 1
PAIN-CONTROL CLINICS FOR ARTHRITIS

Following is a listing of pain-control clinics, which offer a wide variety of pain-control techniques. Each technique is represented by a number, and explained briefly in this introduction. For your convenience, the clinics are listed by state and city.

1. **Acupuncture**—carefully placed needles, sometimes gently rotated by electricity, help eliminate pain.
2. **Allergy**—tests are made to see if arthritis is the result of an allergy. Diets are provided.
3. **Biofeedback**—A technique that allows the unconscious or involuntary bodily processes to be detected by the senses (usually via a TV-like oscilloscope) so that you can control them consciously.
4. **Chiropractic or osteopathic manipulation**—manipulation and adjustment of body structures to allow normal nerve function.
5. **Homeopathic therapies**—a system of medical practice that treats a disease by the administration of minute doses of a remedy that would, in healthy people, produce symptoms of the disease being treated.
6. **Medication reduction**—evaluating and reducing the dosage of medication, usually simultaneous with offering alternative therapy.

7. **Myotherapy**—treating muscles and "trigger points" to reduce pain.

8. **Naturopathy**—treating a disease by assisting nature to heal, often through massage and manipulation.

9. **Nerve block**—a surgical treatment to stop transmission of the pain message.

10. **Neurological treatments**—center on reducing or eliminating the transmission of pain, rather than treating the disease causing the pain. These treatments may include surgery such as nerve blocks.

11. **Nutrition**—therapy for weight loss or vitamin and mineral supplements to the diet to help the body counter disease and heal itself.

12. **Occupational therapy**—offers protection techniques and instruction on how to best perform tasks at work or at home.

13,14. **Pharmacological treatments**—provide **prescription** and **nonprescription drugs (13)**, and **vitamin therapy (14)**.

15. **Physical therapy**—can include specific exercises, hydrotherapy, ultrasound, and massage treatments.

16. **Psychological counseling**—can include a wide variety of treatments, ranging from family and marriage counseling to behavior modification. Some centers also offer psychotherapy.

17. **Relaxation techniques**—can include stress management, yoga, guided visualization, progressive relaxation, and autogenics.

18. **Self-help group therapy**—where others with arthritis offer tips on coping physically and emotionally.

19. **Surgical treatments**—can include orthopedic rehabilitation, nerve blocks, and joint replacements.

20. **Transcutaneous Electrical Nerve Stimulation (TENS)**—a treatment whereby pain transmission is "short-circuited" by a small electrical device.

21. Weight control—to reduce stress on the weight-bearing joints.

ALABAMA
  BIRMINGHAM
    Multi-Purpose Arthritis
      Center
    University Station
    35294
    (205) 934-2130
    (205) 934-2663
    Treatments: 13, 14, 16, 17
    Inpatient and outpatient
    Referral required for inpatient
      treatment only

  BIRMINGHAM
    Pain Center
    University of Alabama-
      Birmingham Medical
      Center
    1920 Seventh Ave., South
    35233
    (205) 934-6174
    Treatments: 1, 3, 11, 12,
    14, 16, 18, 20
    Inpatient and outpatient
    Referral required

ARIZONA
  PHOENIX
    A.R.E. Clinic
    4018 N. Fortieth St.
    85018
    (602) 955-0551
    Treatments: 3, 8, 12, 16, 18
    Outpatient only
    Referral required

  TUCSON
    Pain Clinic
    Arizona Health Sciences
      Center
    University of Arizona
    85724

(602) 626-6239
Treatments: 1, 3, 8, 14, 16,
18
Outpatient only
Referral required

CALIFORNIA
  ALHAMBRA
    New Hope Pain Center
    University of Southern
      California School of
      Medicine
    100 S. Raymond Ave.
    91801
    (213) 570-1607
    Treatments: 3, 10, 11, 13,
    14, 16, 17, 18
    Inpatient and outpatient
    Referral required

  BERKELEY
    Gladman Center
    Hotel Claremont
    41 Tunnel Rd.
    94705
    (415) 549-1228
    Treatments: 3, 12, 17, 18
    Outpatient only
    Referral not required

  BOLINAS
    Commonweal Clinic
    451 Mesa Rd.
    94924
    (415) 868-1501
    Treatments: 11, 12, 18
    Outpatient only
    Referral not required

DESERT HOT SPRINGS
National Arthritis Medical
  Clinic
13-630 Mountain View Rd.
92240
(714) 329-6422
Treatments: 1, 12, 15, 16, 20
Outpatient only
Referral not required

FRESNO
Shu-Ying Lee Medical
  Corporation
3004A N. Fresno St.
93703
(209) 226-4820
Treatment: 1
Outpatient only
Referral required

INGLEWOOD
Centinela Pain Management
  Center
Centinela Hospital Medical
  Center
625 E. Hardy St.
Suite 2
90301
(213) 673-4660
(213) 673-6330
Treatments: 1, 3, 10, 11,
14, 16, 18
Inpatient and outpatient
Referral required

INGLEWOOD
Pain Management Program
Daniel Freeman Hospital
  Medical Center
333 N. Prairie Ave.
90301
(213) 674-7050, ext. 3465
Treatments: 3, 7, 13, 14,
17, 18, 21
Inpatient and outpatient
Referral required

LA JOLLA
Scripps Clinic and Research
  Foundation
10666 N. Torrey Pines Rd.
92037
(714) 455-8898
Treatments: 3, 11, 12, 14,
16, 17, 18, 20, 21
Inpatient and outpatient
Referral required

LOMA LINDA
Pain Control and Health
  Support Services
Loma Linda University
  Medical Center
11375 Anderson St.
92354
(714) 796-0231
Treatments: 1, 3, 10, 14,
16, 18, 21
Outpatient only
Referral required

LONG BEACH
Belvue Medical Clinic
3816 Woodruff Ave.
90808
(213) 420-2611
Treatments: 1, 16, 18
Inpatient and outpatient
Referral required

LOS ANGELES
Bresler Center Medical
  Group
12401 Wilshire Blvd.
Suite 280
90025
(213) 826-5669
Treatments: 1, 3, 4, 11, 12,
16, 17, 18
Outpatient only
Referral not required

LOS ANGELES
  Pain Management Center
  UCLA School of Medicine
  Department of
    Anesthesiology
  10833 La Conte Ave.
  90024
  (213) 825-4291
  Treatments: 1, 3, 8, 10, 11,
  12, 14, 16, 18, 20
  Inpatient and outpatient
  Referral required

SAN DIEGO
  Center for Holistic Health
  4501 Mission Bay Dr.
  92109
  (714) 276-8223
  Treatments: 1, 3, 14, 16, 18
  Outpatient only
  Referral not required

SAN DIEGO
  Orthopedic Rehabilitation
    Clinic
  Rheumatology Clinic
  Pain Clinic
  University Hospital
  225 Dickinson St.
  92103
  (714) 294-6312
  (714) 294-6222
  (714) 294-5899
  Treatments: 11, 12, 14, 16,
  18, 20
  Inpatient and outpatient
  Referral required

COLORADO
  DENVER
    Denver Acupuncture Pain
      Clinic
    350 Cherry Terrace Medical
      Building

3865 N. Cherry Creek
80209
(303) 321-3594
Treatments: 1, 12, 14, 16
Inpatient only
Referral not required

CONNECTICUT
  MIDDLEBURY
    Sung J. Liao, M.D. (Private
      Practice)
    Route 188 and N. Benson Rd.
    06762
    (203) 758-1758
    Treatments: 1, 16
    Outpatient only
    Referral not required

  WATERBURY
    Kent E. Sharian, M.D.
      (Private Practice)
    1389 W. Main St.
    06708
    (203) 753-7900
    Treatments: 1, 3, 12, 14,
    16, 18, 22
    Inpatient and outpatient
    Referral not required

FLORIDA
  MIAMI
    Pain and Back Rehabilitation
      Program
    Department of Neurological
      Surgery D4-6
    University of Miami School
      of Medicine
    P.O. Box 016960
    33101
    (305) 547-6946
    Treatments: 3, 8, 11, 12,
    13, 14, 16, 18, 20
    Inpatient and outpatient
    Referral not required

MIAMI BEACH
  Medical Center Sunny Isles
  Department of Holistic
    Medicine
  18600 Collins Ave.
  33160
  (305) 931-8484
  Treatments: 1, 2, 3, 4, 5, 6,
  8, 10, 11, 12, 14, 16, 17,
  18, 20, 21
  Inpatient and outpatient
  Referral not required

MIAMI BEACH
  The Pain Center
  Mount Sinai Medical Center
  4300 Alton Rd.
  33140
  (305) 674-2070
  Treatments: 1, 10, 11, 14,
  16, 18
  Outpatient only
  Referral not required

NORTH MIAMI
  The Dale Institute for
    Personal and Social Health
  The (W)holistic Treatment
    Center
  The Acupuncture Education
    Center
  13757 Northeast Third Court
  Suite 210A North
  33161
  (305) 891-0062
  (305) 891-7333
  Ralph Alan Dale, Ed.D.,
    Ph.D.—Director
  Treatments: 1, 12, 18
  Outpatient only
  Referral not required
  Open from November to May

NORTH MIAMI BEACH
  The Pain Center
  909 N. Miami Beach Blvd.
  Suite 402
  33162
  (305) 949-6331
  Robert E. Willner, M.D.—
    Director
  Treatments: 1, 6, 8, 11, 12,
  16, 18, 21, 22
  Outpatient only
  Referral not required

GEORGIA
ATLANTA
  Pain Control Center
  Emory University
  1441 Clifton Rd., Northeast
  30322
  (404) 329-5492
  Treatments: 1, 3, 10, 13,
  16, 18, 21
  Inpatient and outpatient
  Referral required

ATLANTA
  Peachtree Pain Clinic
  384 Peachtree St.
  Suite 212
  30308
  (404) 223-5506
  Treatments: 1, 3, 8, 10, 11,
  12, 14, 16, 18, 21
  Outpatient only
  Referral not required

EASTMAN
  Eastman Acupuncture Clinic
  702 Second Ave., West
  31023
  (912) 374-5511
  Channing S. Jun, M.D.—
    Director
  Treatment: 1
  Outpatient only
  Referral not required

IDAHO
　HAMPA
　　John O. Boxall, M.D. (Private
　　　Practice)
　　824 Seventeenth Ave., South
　　83651
　　(208) 466-3518
　　Treatments: 1, 6, 14, 16, 18
　　Outpatient only
　　Referral not required

ILLINOIS
　CHICAGO
　　Arthritis Center
　　Chicago Osteopathic
　　　Hospital
　　5200 S. Ellis
　　60615
　　(312) 947-4998
　　Treatments: 3, 11, 13, 14,
　　16, 18, 20
　　Inpatient and outpatient
　　Referral not required

　CHICAGO
　　Arthritis Clinic
　　Northwestern University
　　　Medical Center
　　222 E. Superior
　　60611
　　(312) 649-8628
　　Treatments: 3, 12, 13, 14,
　　16, 18, 20
　　Inpatient and outpatient
　　Referral required

　CHICAGO
　　Northwest Hospital Pain
　　　Clinic
　　5645 W. Addison St.
　　60634
　　(312) 282-7000
　　Treatments: 1, 10, 11, 14,
　　16, 20, 21
　　Inpatient and outpatient
　　Referral not required

CHICAGO
　Pediatric Pain Clinic
　Children's Memorial Hospital
　Northwestern University
　　Medical School
　2300 Children's Plaza
　60614
　(312) 880-4373
　Treatments: 3, 11, 14, 16,
　18, 20
　Inpatient and outpatient
　Referral not required

CHICAGO
　Rheumatology Clinic
　Cungo Hospital
　750 W. Montrose
　60613
　(312) 883-8149
　Treatments: 11, 12, 14, 16,
　18
　Inpatient and outpatient
　Referral not required

CHICAGO
　Rush Pain Center
　Rush-Presbyterian-St. Luke's
　　Medical Center
　1725 W. Harrison St.
　60612
　(312) 942-6631
　Treatments: 1, 10, 11, 14, 21
　Inpatient and outpatient
　Referral not required

CHICAGO
　St. Joseph Clinic
　2900 N. Lake Shore Dr.
　60657
　(312) 975-3080
　Treatments: 11, 12, 14, 16,
　20
　Inpatient and outpatient
　Referral not required

OLYMPIA FIELDS
Arthritis Center
Olympia Fields Osteopathic
Hospital
20201 S. Crawford
60461
(312) 747-4000, ext. 1156
Treatments: 3, 4, 11, 13,
14, 16, 18, 20, 21
Inpatient and outpatient
Referral not required

PEORIA
Pain Management Clinic
Methodist Medical Center of
Illinois
221 Northeast Glen Oak
61636
(309) 672-5950
Treatments: 3, 8, 10, 12,
14, 16, 18
Inpatient and outpatient
Referral required

ROCKFORD
Chronic Pain Program
Van Matre Rehabilitation
Center
2400 N. Rockton Ave.
61103
(815) 968-6861
Treatments: 3, 8, 12, 13,
14, 16, 17, 18
Inpatient and outpatient
Referral required

IOWA
DES MOINES
Mercy Pain Center
Mercy Medical Center
Sixth and University
50314
(515) 247-3121
Treatments: 3, 6, 11, 12,
15, 16, 21
Inpatient and outpatient
Referral not required

DES MOINES
Steve R. Eckstat, D. O.
(Private Practice)
Mercy Medical Plaza
421 Laurel
Suite 410
50314
(515) 282-8131
Treatments: 3, 12, 14, 15, 16
Inpatient and outpatient
Referral not required

IOWA CITY
Rheumatology Clinic
University of Iowa Hospitals
and Clinics
52240
(319) 356-2413
Treatments: 1, 3, 11, 12,
13, 14, 16, 20
Inpatient and outpatient
Referral required

MAINE
GARDINER
W. M. Tsao, M.D. (Private
Practice)
Acupuncture Clinic
50 Dresden Ave.
04345
(207) 582-2004
Treatment: 1
Outpatient only
Referral not required

MARYLAND
BALTIMORE
Mensana Clinic
Greenspring Valley Road
Stevenson
21153
(301) 653-2403
Treatments: 3, 8, 11, 14,
16, 17, 20, 21
Inpatient and outpatient
Referral required

BALTIMORE
  Pain Treatment Center
  Johns Hopkins Hospital
  601 N. Broadway
  Blalock Building 1404
  21205
  (301) 955-6405
  Treatments: 3, 7, 11, 12, 14,
  16, 18, 20
  Inpatient only
  Referral required

MASSACHUSETTS
  BOSTON
    Adolescent Arthritis Clinic
    Adult Arthritis Clinic
    Pediatric Arthritis Clinic
    New England Medical Center
    171 Harrison Ave.
    02111
    (617) 956-5789
    Treatments: 3, 8, 11, 12,
    13, 14, 16, 18, 20
    Inpatient and outpatient
    Referral not required

  BOSTON
    Lupus Clinic
    Brigham and Women's
      Hospital
    75 Francis St.
    02115
    (617) 732-5350
    Treatments: 3, 14, 16
    Inpatient and outpatient
    Referral not required

  NEW BEDFORD
    Acupuncture Association of
      New Bedford
    1160 Rockdale Ave.
    02740
    (617) 996-5556
    Treatment: 1
    Outpatient only
    Referral not required

WORCESTER
  Pain Control Center
  University of Massachusetts
    Medical Center
  01605
  (617) 856-2640
  Treatments: 3, 10, 12, 14,
  16, 18, 19, 20, 21
  Outpatient only
  Referral required

MICHIGAN
  FARMINGTON
    Farmington Clinic
    24300 Orchard Lake Rd.
    48018
    (313) 474-5601
    Treatments: 1, 12, 14, 16,
    18
    Outpatient only
    Referral not required

  GREENVILLE
    J. Malcolm Nutt, D.O.
      (Private Practice)
    420 S. Lafayette
    48838
    (616) 754-3679
    Treatments: 1, 8, 12, 14
    Outpatient only
    Referral not required

  SOUTHFIELD
    Detroit Pain Clinic
    30003 Southfield
    48076
    (313) 646-8490
    Treatments: 1, 10, 11, 14, 17
    Outpatient only
    Referral not required

MINNESOTA
  HIBBING
    Acupuncture and Pain Clinic
    Central Mesabi Medical
      Center

750 E. Thirty-fourth St.
55746
(218) 262-4881
William C. Lee, M.D.—
  Medical Director
Treatments: 1, 11, 14
Inpatient and outpatient
Referral not required

MINNEAPOLIS
  Acupuncture Clinic
  Mount Sinai Hospital
  2215 Park Ave., South
  55404
  (612) 871-3700, ext. 1248
  Treatments: 1, 10
  Inpatient and outpatient
  Referral required

MINNEAPOLIS
  Rheumatology Clinic
  Mayo Memorial Building
  University of Minnesota
  420 Delaware St., Southeast
  55455
  (612) 376-8613
  Treatments: 1, 8, 11, 12,
  14, 16, 18, 20
  Inpatient and outpatient
  Referral not required

ROCHESTER
  Pain Clinic
  Mayo Clinic
  200 First St., Southwest
  55901
  (507) 284-8311
  Treatments: 1, 3, 10, 11,
  14, 16, 18, 20, 21
  Outpatient only
  Referral required

ROCHESTER
  Pain Management Center
  Mayo Clinic

1216 Second St., Southwest
  and 200 First St.,
  Southwest
55901
(507) 284-2933
Treatments: 3, 16, 17, 18
Inpatient only
Referral required

MISSOURI
  SPRINGFIELD
    Shealy Pain and Health
      Rehabilitation Institute
    St. John's Regional Health
      Center
    1919 S. Fremont
    68504
    (417) 882-0850
    Treatments: 1, 3, 8, 11, 12,
    15, 16, 18, 20, 21
    Inpatient and outpatient
    Referral not required

NEBRASKA
  OMAHA
    Nebraska Pain Management
      Center
    University of Nebraska
      Hospital and Clinic
    Forty-second and Dewey Ave.
    68105
    (402) 559-4301
    Treatments: 3, 8, 16, 17, 18
    Inpatient and outpatient
    Referral required

NEVADA
  LAS VEGAS
    Willem H. Khoe, M.D., Ph.D.
      (Private Practice)
    Spring Valley Health Center
    3880 S. Tones
    Suite 214
    89103
    (702) 871-5599

Treatments: 1, 5, 8, 12, 16, 18
Outpatient only
Referral not required

NEW HAMPSHIRE
  MANCHESTER
    Arthritis Clinic
    Outpatient Clinic
    Veterans Administration
      Hospital
    718 Smyth Rd.
    03104
    (603) 624-4366, ext. 379
    Treatments: 3, 11, 14, 16, 18, 20
    Inpatient and outpatient
    Referral required

NEW JERSEY
  IRVINGTON
    Harold E. Lippman, M.D.
      (Private Practice)
    40 Union Ave.
    07111
    (201) 374-1414
    Treatments: 1, 16, 21
    Outpatient only
    Referral not required

  PARAMUS
    Nan-Sung Chu, M.D. (Private
      Practice)
    122 E. Ridgewood Ave.
    07652
    (201) 652-7807
    Treatment: 1
    Outpatient only
    Referral not required

  SOUTH PLAINFIELD
    Mark Friedman, M.D.
      (Private Practice)
    2509 Park Ave.
    07080

(201) 753-8622
Treatments: 1, 3, 8, 11, 12, 14, 16, 17, 18
Inpatient and outpatient
Referral not required

NEW YORK
  EAST MEADOW
    Arthritis Clinic
    Nassau County Medical
      Center
    Hempstead Turnpike
    11554
    (516) 542-0123
    Treatments: 3, 8, 14, 16, 18, 20
    Inpatient and outpatient
    Referral required

  ELMIRA
    Pain Control Program
    Arnot Ogden Memorial
      Hospital
    Roe Ave.
    14901
    (607) 737-4211
    Treatments: 3, 8, 10, 11, 12, 14, 16, 18, 20
    Outpatient only
    Referral required

  FLORAL PARK
    Nassau-Queens Physical
      Medicine and
      Rehabilitation Services
    One Cisney Ave.
    11001
    (516) 354-4045
    Treatments: 1, 3, 6, 8, 11, 13, 14, 16, 18
    Outpatient only
    Referral not required

FLUSHING
Department of Rehabilitation
Medicine
Booth Memorial Medical
Center
5645 Main St.
11355
(212) 670-1290
Treatments: 3, 14, 16, 17,
18, 21
Inpatient and outpatient
Referral required

HAVERSTRAW
Regional Bone Center
Helen Hayes Hospital
Route 9W
10993
(914) 947-3000
Treatments: 11, 12, 14, 16, 18
Inpatient and outpatient
Referral not required

MAMARONECK
Allen L. Chodock, M.D.
(Private Practice)
1600 Harrison Ave.
10543
(914) 698-2902
Treatments: 1, 14, 16
Inpatient and outpatient
Referral not required

MONTOUR FALLS
Acupuncture Research
Center
Schuyler Hospital
14865
(607) 535-7121
Treatments: 1, 16, 20
Inpatient and outpatient
Referral required

NEW YORK CITY (Bronx)
Arthritis Clinic
Misericordia Hospital
Medical Center Clinic
600 E. 233rd St.
10466
(212) 920-9744
Treatments: 11, 12, 14, 16
Inpatient and outpatient
Referral required

NEW YORK CITY (Bronx)
Pain Treatment Center
Montefiore Hospital Medical
Center
111 E. 210th St.
10467
(212) 920-4440
Treatments: 1, 3, 14, 16,
17, 21
Outpatient only
Referral required

NEW YORK CITY (Brooklyn)
Arthritis Clinic
State University of New York
Downstate Medical Center
470 Clarkson Ave.
11203
(212) 270-1321
Treatments: 14, 16, 19, 20
Inpatient and outpatient
Referral not required

NEW YORK CITY (Brooklyn)
Coney Island Acupuncture
Clinic
2802 Mermaid Ave.
11224
(212) 372-4569
Treatments: 1, 3, 6, 12, 18
Outpatient only
Referral not required

NEW YORK CITY (Brooklyn)
Pain Therapy Center
Maimonides Medical Center
931 Forty-eighth St.
11219
(212) 270-7177
(212) 270-7182
Treatments: 1, 3, 10, 11,
14, 16, 18
Outpatient only
Referral required

NEW YORK CITY
(Manhattan)
Acupuncture Treatment
Group of New York
426 E. Eighty-ninth St.
10028
(212) 534-6800
Ralph Sepson, M.D.—
Director
Treatment: 1
Outpatient only
Referral not required

NEW YORK CITY
(Manhattan)
Arthritis Clinic
Mt. Sinai Hospital
One E. 100th St.
10029
(212) 650-6500, ext. 7104
Treatments: 12, 14, 16
Outpatient only
Referral required

NEW YORK CITY
(Manhattan)
Hand Service Institute of
Rehabilitation Medicine
New York University Medical
Center
400 E. Thirty-fourth St.
10016
(212) 340-6098

Don Chu, M.D.—Director
Treatments: 3, 11, 13, 14,
16, 18, 20
Treatment limited to hand
problems only
Inpatient and outpatient
Referral required

NEW YORK CITY
(Manhattan)
Orthopaedic Clinics
Hand Clinic
Hip Clinic
Knee Clinic
Rheumatic Disease Clinic
Sports Medicine Clinic
Hospital for Special Surgery
535 E. Seventieth St.
10021
(212) 535-4555
(212) 535-4556
Treatments: 11, 12, 14, 16, 20
Inpatient and outpatient
Referral not required

NEW YORK CITY
(Manhattan)
Pain Service
Hospital for Joint Diseases
Orthopaedic Institute
301 E. Seventeenth St.
10003
(212) 598-6260
Treatments: 3, 11, 13, 14,
16, 17, 18, 20, 21
Inpatient and outpatient
Referral required

NEW YORK CITY
(Manhattan)
Rheumatic Disease Clinic
Hospital for Special Surgery
535 E. Seventieth St.
10021

(212) 535-4555
(212) 535-4556
Treatments: 11, 12, 13, 14,
16, 20
Inpatient and outpatient
Referral required

NEW YORK CITY
(Manhattan)
Rheumatology Section
Metropolitan Hospital Center
1901 First Ave.
10024
(212) 360-6771
Treatments: 8, 11, 12, 14,
16, 18, 20
Inpatient and outpatient
Referral not required

NEW YORK CITY
(Manhattan)
Daniel S. J. Choy, M.D.
(Private Practice)
170 E. Seventy-seventh St.
10021
(212) 535-6040
Treatments: 1, 14
Outpatient only
Referral not required

NEW YORK CITY
(Manhattan)
Ling Sun Chu, M.D. (Private
Practice)
107 E. Seventy-third St.
10021
(212) 472-3000
Treatments: 1, 14, 16
Outpatient only
Referral not required

NEW YORK CITY
(Manhattan)
Frank Z. Warren, M.D.
(Private Practice)

141 E. Eighty-eighth St.
10028
(212) 427-8390
Treatments: 1, 12, 14, 18
Inpatient and outpatient
Referral not required

NORTH TARRYTOWN
Phelps Pain Clinic
Phelps Memorial Hospital
Center
North Broadway
10591
(914) 631-5100
Treatments: 1, 8, 11, 14,
16, 20
Inpatient and outpatient
Referral required

NORWICH
Acupuncture Clinic
Experimental Medicine and
Research
Chenango Memorial Hospital
R.D. #3, Box 480
13815
(607) 334-9994
Treatment: 1
Inpatient and outpatient
Referral required

PARKSVILLE
The Dale Institute for
Personal and Social Health
The (W)holistic Treatment
Center
The Acupuncture Education
Center
Muhlig Rd.
12768
(914) 292-8080
(914) 292-8050
Ralph Alan Dale, Ed.D.,
Ph.D.—Director
Treatments: 1, 12, 18

Outpatient only
Referral not required
Open from May to November

SYRACUSE
Back Rehabilitation Program
Upstate Medical Center and
   St. Camillus Hospital
813 Fay Rd.
13219
(315) 488-2951, ext. 212
Treatments: 3, 13, 16, 17,
   18, 22
Treatment limited to back
   problems only
Inpatient and outpatient
Referral required

SYRACUSE
Pain Treatment Service
Upstate Medical Center
State University of New York
750 E. Adams St.
13210
(315) 473-4720
Treatments: 1, 3, 8, 14, 16, 18
Outpatient only
Referral required

WHITE PLAINS
Pain Treatment Center
St. Agnes Hospital
305 North St.
10605
(914) 682-3788
Treatments: 1, 3, 6, 8, 10, 11,
   12, 14, 16, 18, 20
Inpatient and outpatient
Referral required

NORTH CAROLINA
CHAPEL HILL
Arthritis Clinic
North Carolina Memorial
   Hospital

Manning Dr.
27514
(919) 966-4191
(919) 966-3017 (Monday,
   Wednesday, Friday)
Treatments: 3, 6, 11, 12,
   13, 14, 16, 17, 18, 20
Inpatient and outpatient
Referral required

DURHAM
Rheumatology Clinic
Duke University Medical
   Center
P.O. Box 3892
27710
(919) 684-6205
Treatments: 3, 14, 16, 20
Inpatient and outpatient
Referral required

WINSTON-SALEM
Rheumatology Clinic
North Carolina Baptist
   Hospital
Bowman Gray School of
   Medicine
300 S. Hawthorne Rd.
27103
(919) 748-4209
Treatments: 3, 14, 16, 18, 20
Inpatient and outpatient
Referral required

OHIO
CINCINNATI
Pain Control Center
University of Cincinnati
   Medical Center
234 Goodman St.
Old Administration Building
45267
(513) 872-5664
Treatments: 1, 3, 6, 10, 11,
   17, 18, 21

Inpatient and outpatient
Referral required

CINCINNATI
Special Treatment Center for
Juvenile Arthritis
Rm. 1-29
Pavilion Building
University of Cincinnati
Children's Hospital Medical
Center
45229
(513) 559-4676
Treatments: 3, 14, 16, 18, 20
Inpatient and outpatient
Referral required

CLEVELAND
Arthritis Clinic
Cleveland Metropolitan
General Hospital
3395 Scranton Rd.
44109
(216) 459-4195
Treatments: 12, 14, 16
Inpatient and outpatient
Referral not required

CLEVELAND
Cleveland Clinic Foundation
9500 Euclid Ave.
44106
(216) 444-5632
Treatments: 3, 11, 12, 14,
16, 18, 20
Inpatient and outpatient
Referral not required

CLEVELAND
Rheumatology Clinic/
Ambulatory Care Center
St. Vincent Charity Hospital
and Health Center
2351 E. Twenty-second St.
44115

(216) 861-6200
Treatments: 13, 16, 17
Inpatient and outpatient
Referral required

CLEVELAND
Jeffrey A. Chaitoff, M.D.
(Private Practice)
14055 Cedar Rd.
44118
(216) 371-3181
Treatments: 11, 12, 14, 16,
21
Outpatient only
Referral not required

COLUMBUS
The Ohio Pain and Stress
Treatment Center
1460 W. Lake Ave.
43221
(614) 488-5971
Treatments: 3, 7, 11, 12, 17,
18
Outpatient only
Referral not required

SOUTH EUCLID
Ambulatory Care Center
University Suburban Health
Center
1611 S. Green Rd.
44121
(216) 382-8920
Treatments: 11, 12, 16, 20
Outpatient only
Referral required

YOUNGSTOWN
James W. Dabney, D.O.
(Private Practice)
Wick Avenue Doctors Clinic
1407 Wick Ave.
44505
(216) 747-5913

Treatment: 1
Outpatient only
Referral not required

OREGON
PORTLAND
Acupuncture Pain Control
Center
7227 Southwest Terwilliger
97219
(503) 245-3156
Treatments: 1, 3, 9, 12, 14,
16, 18
Outpatient only
Referral not required

PORTLAND
Northwest Pain Center
University of Oregon Medical
School
10615 Southeast Cherry
Blossom Dr.
Suite 170
97216
(503) 256-1930
Treatments: 1, 3, 11, 12,
14, 16, 17, 18
Outpatient only
Referral required

PENNSYLVANIA
PHILADELPHIA
Rheumatology Associates
Germantown Hospital
2 Penn Blvd.
19147
(215) 844-1118
Treatments: 3, 14, 16, 20
Inpatient and outpatient
Referral not required

PITTSBURGH
Arthritis Clinic
Children's Hospital
125 DeSota St.

15213
(412) 647-5435
Treatments: 3, 8, 12, 14, 16
Inpatient and outpatient
Referral required

SOUTH CAROLINA
CHARLESTON
Arthritis Center
Medical University of South
Carolina
171 Ashley Ave.
29425
(803) 792-4152
Treatments: 3, 13, 14, 16,
18
Inpatient and outpatient
Referral required

TENNESSEE
MEMPHIS
Pain Clinic
Faculty Medical Practice
Corp., P.C.
66 N. Pauline
38105
(901) 528-6638
Treatments: 3, 10, 11, 14,
16, 18
Inpatient and outpatient
Referral required

TEXAS
DALLAS
Pain Evaluation and
Treatment Center
University of Texas Health
Science Center
5323 Harry Hines Blvd.
75235
(214) 688-2774
Treatments: 1, 3, 6, 8, 10,
11, 16, 18
Outpatient only
Referral required

DALLAS
R. W. Noble, M.D. (Private
Practice)
115 W. Preston Forest Village
75230
(214) 368-1403
Treatments: 2, 12, 14, 16
Outpatient only
Referral not required

HOUSTON
University of Texas Pain
Clinic
Houston/Hermann Hospital
6431 Fannin St.
MSMB 7148
77030
(713) 792-5760
Treatments: 3, 11, 14, 16,
17, 18, 20
Inpatient and outpatient
Referral required

IRVING
Irving Medical Center, P.A.
620 N. O'Connor
75060
(214) 259-3541
Treatments: 1, 3, 8, 10, 11,
12, 14, 16, 18
Outpatient only
Referral not required

SAN ANTONIO
Arthritis Clinic of San
Antonio
Metropolitan Professional
Building
1310 McCullough St.
78212
(512) 224-4421
Treatments: 8, 14, 16, 18
Inpatient and outpatient
Referral not required

UTAH
OGDEN
Jeffrey E. Booth, M.D.
(Private Practice)
3905 Harrison Blvd.
#508
84403
(801) 399-4431
Treatments: 3, 12, 14, 16,
18
Inpatient and outpatient
Referral not required

SALT LAKE CITY
Salt Lake Clinic
Latter Day Saints Hospital
333 S. Ninth, East
84102
(801) 535-8182
Treatments: 3, 8, 12, 14,
16, 18, 20
Inpatient and outpatient
Referral not required

VERMONT
WHITE RIVER JUNCTION
Arthritis Clinic
Veterans Administration
Hospital
N. Heartland
05001
(802) 295-9363
Treatments: 3, 11, 13, 14,
16, 17, 18, 20
Inpatient and outpatient
Referral required

VIRGINIA
CHARLOTTESVILLE
Department of
Anesthesiology Pain Clinic
University of Virginia
Box 293
22908
(804) 924-5581

Treatments: 3, 8, 10, 11, 12, 14, 16, 17, 18, 21
Outpatient only
Referral required

WASHINGTON
  SEATTLE
  Children's Arthritis Clinic
  Children's Orthopedic
    Hospital and Medical
    Center
  University of Washington
  4800 Sand Point Way,
    Northeast
  98105
  (206) 634-5512
  Treatments: 3, 13, 14, 16, 20
  Inpatient and outpatient
  Referral not required

  SEATTLE
  Clinical Pain Service
  University of Washington
    Medical School
  Northeast Pacific
  98195
  (206) 543-3236
  Treatments: 1, 3, 10, 11, 12, 14, 16, 18, 20
  Inpatient and outpatient
  Referral required

  SEATTLE
  R. N. Toynea, Jr., M.D.
    (Private Practice)
  2041 E. Madison St.
  98122
  (206) 722-2668
  Treatments: 1, 14, 16
  Outpatient only
  Referral not required

  SPOKANE
  Empire Medical Clinic
  E17 Empire

99207
(509) 328-3430
Treatments: 1, 8, 12, 14
Outpatient only
Referral not required

  TACOMA
  J. Hugh Kalkus, M.D.
    (Private Practice)
  Fife Medical Office
  5619 Valley Ave., East
  98424
  (206) 922-0311
  Treatments: 1, 6, 14, 18
  Inpatient only
  Referral not required

WEST VIRGINIA
  MORGANTOWN
  Pain Clinic
  West Virginia University
    Medical Center
  26506
  (304) 293-5411
  Treatments: 3, 8, 10, 11, 12, 14, 16, 18, 21, 22
  Inpatient and outpatient
  Referral required

  MORGANTOWN
  Rheumatology Clinic
  West Virginia University
    Medical Center
  26506
  (304) 293-4901
  Treatments: 3, 11, 12, 14, 16, 18
  Inpatient and outpatient
  Referral not required

WISCONSIN
  MADISON
  Lakeview Medical Clinic S.C.
  2830 Dryden Dr.
  53704

(608) 241-3451
Treatments: 1, 4, 16
Outpatient only
Referral not required

MADISON
Pain Clinic
University of Wisconsin
600 Highland Ave.
53792
(608) 263-8094
Treatments: 3, 10, 11, 14,
16, 18, 20, 21
Inpatient and outpatient
Referral required

MILWAUKEE
Pain Management Clinic
Curative Rehabilitation
  Center
9001 W. Watertown Plank Rd.
53226
(414) 259-1414
Treatments: 3, 8, 13, 16,
17, 18
Outpatient only
Referral required

MANITOBA (Canada)
WINNIPEG
Acupuncture Research
  Foundation of Manitoba
Victoria General Hospital
640 Broadway Ave.
R3C 0X3
(204) 774-2385
Treatments: 1, 8, 11, 14,
16, 18
Inpatient and outpatient
Referral required

WINNIPEG
Pain Clinic
Victoria General Hospital
2340 Pembino Highway
R3T 2E8
(204) 269-3570
Treatments: 1, 3, 11, 14,
16, 18
Inpatient and outpatient
Referral not required

Appendix 2

A GLOSSARY OF ARTHRITIS TERMINOLOGY

acupressure   pressing on the acupuncture points that normally would be pricked with a needle in an effort to relieve pain.

acupuncture   the Chinese practice of inserting needles into specific points along the "meridians" of the body to relieve the discomfort associated with painful disorders, to induce surgical anesthesia, and for preventive and therapeutic purposes.

adaptive immunity   recognition and differentiation of foreign matter from the body's own material.

adrenal cortex   the outer shell of the adrenal gland.

adrenal glands   two small glands which are located on top of the kidneys.

analgesic   a drug that relieves pain.

ankylosing spondylitis   a fairly common form of arthritis which primarily affects men but also strikes women; characterized by cycles of pain and stiffness in the lower back.

ankylosis   abnormal immobility and consolidation of a joint.

antigen   any substance which can bring about the formation of an antibody.

aplastic anemia   a form of bone marrow failure which impairs the production of all three types of blood cells produced by the bone marrow.

arrhythmia   variation from the normal rhythm, especially of the heartbeat.

arthrodesis   a surgical procedure designed to produce fusion of a joint.

arthropathy   a disease affecting a joint.

arthroplasty   any surgical procedure that reconstructs a joint; may or may not involve an artificial replacement.

arthroscope   an instrument for examining the inside of a joint.

arthrosis   a disease limited to cartilage degeneration with no joint inflammation.

articular   of or pertaining to a joint.

atrophy   a decrease in the size of a normally developed organ or tissue; wasting away.

autoimmune   a malfunction of the body's immune system
  disease   whereby cells filled with digestive enzymes destroy what they believe is foreign matter.

autonomic   the branch of the nervous system that works
  nervous   without conscious control; affects such functions
  system   as heart rate and digestion and plays a critical role in the relief of chronic pain.

Baker's cyst   a cyst or swelling behind the knee, causing an accumulation of fluid in the bursae.

bamboo spine — a descriptive term for the appearance of the spine in ankylosing spondylitis.

bioelectricity — the electrical energy that appears in living tissue, generated by the muscles and nerves.

blood count — one of the most common tests done on the blood; it represents the number of blood cells in a given sample of blood, usually expressed as the number of cells in a cubic millimeter of blood.

bone marrow depression — a serious reduction in the ability of the bone marrow to produce red blood cells, white blood cells, or blood platelets; blood examinations can reveal specific changes in the level of each type.

bony spurs (osteophytes) — a pointed projection of bone.

bunion — an inflamed swelling of a small sac on the first joint of the big toe.

bursa — a little pouch containing a gummy fluid used to lubricate body tissues which have to rub against one another.

bursitis — inflammation of a small sac, found near a joint, which provides lubrication.

calcific tendinitis — inflammation of a tendon, usually caused by calcium deposits.

carboxylic acid — a class of organic acids that includes fatty acids, salicylates, and amino acids.

carpal tunnel syndrome — a type of tenosynovitis which causes pain in the wrist, fingers, and forearm; characterized by an accumulation of fluid inside the carpal tunnel that puts pressure on the nerve that makes it possible for you to move your fingers.

carrier effect the ability of one substance to move a second substance along with it through a membrane.

chelation a process by which a chemical combines with a metal that is naturally present in the body.

chi Chinese term for the vital energy flow or life force which circulates through the body along meridians.

Chinese restaurant syndrome may appear about 20 minutes after eating a meal spiced heavily with monosodium glutamate (MSG); includes headache, feverish flush, and a detached feeling.

chondrocalcinosis a condition which usually attacks older people; caused when crystals made of calcium salts gradually develop and gravitate to the larger joints, especially the knee.

chronic rheumatoid arthritis a form of arthritis, the cause of which is unknown, although infection, hypersensitivity, hormone imbalance, and psychologic stress have been suggested as possible causes; a state which persists for a long time and shows little change or extremely slow progress.

chronic tophaceous gout the fourth stage of gout where the attacks come and stay with the person; characterized by chalky deposits on the body's bony knobs.

colitis inflammation of the colon; may be accompanied by cramplike pain in the upper stomach, and constipation sometimes alternating with diarrhea.

collagen a fiberlike protein substance.

conjunctivae the delicate membrane lining the eyelids and covering the eyeball.

connective tissue a general term used to describe tissue that connects one part of the body to another; includes fibrous tissue, bone, cartilage, synovium, blood vessels, ligaments, tendons, and parts of muscle.

contrast baths a treatment used to increase blood flow to the extremities to help healing and eliminating pain; involves placing hands and feet in hot water, then cold.

cortisone a hormone produced in the body by the adrenal glands; has also been synthesized in the laboratory and used as a drug.

Crohn's disease inflammation of the last portion of the small intestine; called also regional enteritis and regional ileitis.

cytotoxic food allergy test a testing method that measures the reaction of a person's white blood cells to a particular food; the degree of destruction of the white blood cells theoretically will pinpoint foods to which a person is allergic.

degenerative joint disease a noninflammatory, slowly progressive disorder of joints caused by deterioration of articular cartilage, followed by bone formation.

diathermy the use of high-frequency electrical currents as a form of physical therapy and in surgical procedures.

DMSO (dimethyl sulfoxide) a by-product of wood pulp manufacture which is known for its "carrying ability," and which some believe relieves joint pain.

double-blind crossover technique a situation where neither the patients nor the doctors conducting an experiment know which patients receive the actual test substance and which receive the placebo.

dysfunctional pain an abnormal function of muscles and joints which causes instant pain and allows limited mobility.

edema accumulation of excess fluid in the tissues (swelling).

EEG (electro-encephalo-gram) a tracing of the electrical impulses of the brain.

effusion excess fluid in the joint indicating irritation or inflammation of the synovium.

EKG (electro-cardio-gram) a tracing representing the heart's electrical action derived by amplification of the minutely small electrical impulses normally generated by the heart.

endorphins natural painkillers released by the brain.

epithelial cells cells joined by small amounts of cementing substances; they cover internal and external surfaces of the body, including the lining of vessels and other small cavities.

erythema redness.

gate theory proposes that if you overload certain nerve fibers with sensations other than pain, you can block the pain message from reaching the brain.

gout a disease characterized by acute episodes of arthritis with the presence of sodium urate crystals in the synovial fluid or deposits of urate crystals in or about the joints and other tissues.

Heberden's nodes the bony knobs that show up at the end joints of the fingers.

hepatitis inflammation of the liver.

HLA-B27   an antigen found in the blood of persons who have
                       the B27 gene for a particular tissue type; used to
                       diagnose arthritis, especially ankylosing spon-
                       dylitis.

Hubbard tank   a huge tank, shaped like a figure eight, with
                       pulleys, straps, and levers that lower a person
                       into and out of water; used for hydrotherapy.

**hydrogym-   exercises done in water which improve muscle
   nastics**   strength, balance, and coordination.

hydrotherapy   a water treatment used to relieve symptoms for
                       any kind of arthritis.

hypercalciuria   excess of calcium in the urine.

**hyperpara-   overactive parathyroid glands, causing loss of cal-
   thyroidism**   cium from the bones and excessive secretion of
                       calcium and phosphorus by the kidneys.

hyperthermia   an abnormally high body temperature sometimes
                       used for therapeutic purposes.

**hypertrophic   another term for degenerative joint disease.
   arthritis**

hyperuricemia   a precondition of gout where there is a growing
                       level of uric acid in the blood.

iatrogenic   caused by inappropriate medical treatment.

**immuno-   a substance that enhances the efficiency of the
   stimulant**   immune system.

**inborn error of   a hereditary biochemical disorder in which a spe-
   metabolism**   cific enzyme defect produces a metabolic prob-
                       lem that may cause disease.

innate immunity   instantaneous recognition and destruction of for-
                       eign matter by the body's immune system.

interstitial   a rare and painful bladder disease.
  cystitis

iritis   inflammation of the iris and the area surrounding
                          it, typically seen in juvenile rheumatoid arthritis
                          and other rheumatoid diseases; can cause scar-
                          ring and lead to loss of vision.

isometric   exercises involving muscle contraction without
  exercises   joint motion.

jaundice   a symptom of one of a number of different dis-
                          eases and disorders of the liver, gallbladder, and
                          blood which results in a yellowness of skin, white
                          of the eye, and excretions.

joint capsule   the tough, fibrous tissue around the area where
                          the ends of bones meet, are lubricated, and
                          cushioned so that they can slide easily past one
                          another.

joint fluid   an examination of the joint fluid done by inserting
  examination   a needle into the sore joint and withdrawing a few
                          drops of fluid.

joint fusion   freezing of bones together, effectively removing
  (arthro-   the joint.
  desis)

joint mouse   an osteophyte that has broken away from the
                          bone and moves about inside the joint space.

joint replace-   artificial joints substituted for real joints; avail-
  ment   able for the hips, wrists, elbows, shoulders,
                          knees, and fingers.

lumbar   the five vertebrae of the lower back.
  vertebrae

malaise   a feeling of general discomfort or uneasiness.

monocyclic rheumatoid arthritis a basic pattern of rheumatoid arthritis in which symptoms last for a few months, then disappear.

myalgia muscle pain.

myasthenia gravis a chronic disease characterized by muscular weakness, caused by a chemical defect at the site where the nerves and muscles interact.

myelin the protective sheath that surrounds nerve fibers.

myotherapy muscle treatments to reduce pain that include massage, ultrasound, or pressure applied to "trigger points."

older onset juvenile rheumatoid arthritis a type of pauciarticular juvenile rheumatoid arthritis which hits children 8 years or older.

ostectomy (osteotomy) surgically cutting a bone.

osteopenia any condition involving reduced bone mass.

osteophytes bony spurs that develop during the course of osteoarthritis.

osteoporosis a condition characterized by a loss of bone cells; can be a disease that comes on by itself, or develops as a result of other diseases, drug therapies, or disuse; can be improved or minimized with active motion and exercise.

pannus a shaggy growth resulting from the unchecked invasion of the synovial tissue into the joint space.

passive exercise exercise where another person or a machine provides the muscle.

pauciarticular juvenile rheumatoid arthritis   the mildest form of juvenile rheumatoid arthritis which affects only one or two joints but which can also cause a disease of the iris; affects people under age 16.

peripheral arthritis   a type of arthritis occurring infrequently and characterized by a sudden onset which affects the knees and ankles and possibly other joints.

phlebitis   inflammation of a vein.

placebo   an inactive substance or preparation given to satisfy the patient's need for drug therapy; also used in scientific studies to determine the effectiveness of medicinal substances.

podagra   a type of gout which attacks the big toe.

polyarticular juvenile rheumatoid arthritis   a type of childhood juvenile rheumatoid arthritis which usually affects four or more joints, causes a low-grade fever, nodules under the skin, and sometimes anemia.

polycyclic rheumatoid arthritis   a pattern of rheumatoid arthritis in which symptoms come in a series of attacks but leaves you feeling well between bouts.

postural pain   a type of pain which comes on gradually, is relieved by stretching or changing position; causes a person to wake up stiff and sore but with full mobility.

primary osteoarthritis   a type of degenerative joint disease where stiffness occurs with no apparent cause.

prostaglandins   a group of fatty acids produced throughout the body and released when cells have been damaged.

pseudogout   a condition that closely resembles gout but which has a different cause; also called chondrocalcinosis.

quantitative   based on a total amount or number; involving a measurement of an amount.

range of motion (ROM)   exercises that move each joint through the full range of motion, that is, to the highest degree of motion of which each joint normally is capable.

regional enteritis   inflammation of the last portion of the small intestine; called also regional ileitis or Crohn's disease.

Reiter's disease   a rare form of arthritis associated with inflammatory bowel disease; assumed to be a result of infectious bacteria; not only affects the joints but also the genitals and the eyes.

Rheumatoid Factor test (RF)   a blood test that searches specifically for a rheumatoid factor circulating in the blood.

sacroiliac   the joint in the lower back where the little triangular bone just above the buttocks meets the hip bones.

scleroderma   a chronic disorder characterized by progressive hardening and shrinking of the connective tissue in many organs and systems, usually beginning with the skin.

scurvy   a deficiency disease caused by a lack of vitamin C; results in blood collecting in the body's joints, causing them to become stiff and painful.

secondary osteoarthritis   a type of degenerative joint disease where stiffness occurs from a clearly identifiable problem.

sedimentation rate   the rate at which red blood cells settle in the blood's serum; elevated in any inflammatory disease such as rheumatoid arthritis.

sedimentation rate test a blood test used to indicate the degree of inflammation in a person's joints; it measures the speed at which red blood cells will settle from whole, unclotted blood; in general, the slower the cells settle, the less chance there is of disease or the greater the degree of improvement.

slipped disk a popular name for a rupture of a disk, or pad of cartilage, between vertebrae.

subluxation incomplete or partial dislocation.

synovectomy a surgical procedure to remove the synovial membrane.

synovial membrane the membrane that surrounds the joint and provides the joint's lubricating fluid.

synovitis inflammation of the synovial membrane.

systemic juvenile rheumatoid arthritis a type of childhood juvenile rheumatoid arthritis which can hit any number of joints or just one, and is usually accompanied by a high fever, salmon-colored rash, irritation of the iris, enlargement of the liver and spleen, and pain in the upper spine.

tendinitis inflammation of the tendon, the tough cord that leads from the muscle to the joint.

tenosynovitis a condition where joint pain arises because of an inflammation of the tube through which the tendon passes.

tinnitus persistent ringing or buzzing in the ears used as an indicator of aspirin toxicity.

tophi growths that appear over the body's bony knobs or along the outer edges of the ears; made of sodium urate crystals.

TENS (transcu-
taneous
electrical
nerve
stimulation) therapy that uses electrical currents running through electrodes attached to the skin; these electrical messages spur the brain to produce higher than normal amounts of endorphins and other body-produced painkillers.

ulcerative colitis a chronic ulceration in the colon producing diarrhea, loss of weight, and sometimes anemia.

uricosuric agent slows down the absorption of uric acid salts by the kidneys, thus increasing the amount of uric acid you excrete and decreasing the amount in your blood.

urinalysis analysis of the urine to determine whether it contains abnormal substances indicative of disease.

varicose veins swollen, distended, and knotted veins, usually found in the legs; result from a stagnated or sluggish flow of the blood, in combination with defective valves and weakened walls of the veins.

Wilson's disease a hereditary disorder of copper metabolism.

young onset
juvenile
rheumatoid
arthritis a type of pauciarticular juvenile rheumatoid arthritis which hits children 5 years old or younger.

_____ Appendix 3 _____
ARTHRITIS DRUGS: SIDE EFFECTS, INTERACTIONS, AND COSTS

Brand Name/ Generic Name	Benefits and/ or Uses	Side Effects[1]

ASPIRIN OR ASPIRINLIKE ARTHRITIS DRUGS

| **All Brands**
aspirin (acetyl-
salicylic acid)
and buffered
aspirin | Analgesic
Anti-inflam-
matory
Used for all
types of arthritis | High doses (10–
15 tablets per
day) can cause
gastrointestinal
problems includ-
ing sour stom-
ach, nausea,
vomiting, ulcers,
and intestinal
bleeding.

Less common
are ringing in the
ears and hearing
loss, painful red-
violet swelling of
the skin, rapid |

SOURCES: Adapted from *Hazards of Medication,* 2d ed., by Eric W. Martin et al. (Phila-delphia: J. B. Lippincott, 1978).

Martindale, The Extra Pharmacopoeia, 27th ed. Ainley Wade, ed. (London: Pharmaceutical Press, 1977).

Physicians' Desk Reference, 36th ed. (Oradell, N.J.: Medical Economics, 1982).

Physicians' Desk Reference for Nonprescription Drugs, 2d ed. (Oradell, N.J.: Medical Economics, 1981).

The Essential Guide to Prescription Drugs, by James W. Long (New York: Harper and Row, 1982).

The Physicians' Drug Manual, Rubin Bressler et al., eds. (Garden City, N.Y.: Doubleday and Co., 1981).

NOTES: Information in this table should be considered informative and not prescriptive or all-encompassing.

Costs reflect prices in the Allentown, Pennsylvania, area in September, 1982. Prices in other areas may vary.

Drugs are listed in the order of how may people use them, with the most commonly used (aspirin) at the beginning and the least commonly used at the end.

Interactions and Precautions[2]	Average Costs[3],[4] (Drug, Lab, etc.)

Probenecid, sulfinpyrazone, and phenylbutazone have decreased effects when taken with salicylates.	$8.95–$15.70
Alcohol, corticosteriods, oxyphenbutazone, and phenylbutazone increase the risk of gastrointestinal ulcer.	
Corticosteroids enhance irritation of the stomach, leading to ulceration.	
Aspirin increases blood clotting time, which interferes with the effects of anticoagulants.	
Aspirin increases the rate of excretion of vitamin C in the urine, which, in turn, decreases the excretion of aspirin, enhancing its activity.	

1. Every individual may react to each of these drugs differently. Some side effects are unavoidable and not dangerous (only annoying). Others, such as aplastic anemia, are dangerous and even fatal. If you are affected by any of these side effects, check with your doctor.
2. Drug interactions that cause increased or decreased effectiveness of either drug will affect drug dosages and the risk of toxicity. See your physician for dosage adjustments.
3. Prices listed are averages based on suggested dosage. They may vary with dose, region, or even individual pharmacy.
4. Costs are based on a one-month treatment period unless otherwise noted.
5. Edema or water retention can cause high blood pressure and be risky for persons with heart problems or hypertension.
6. Prices reflect only the cost of maintenance doses and not the initial treatment costs.
7. Average cost based on a wide range of dosages.
8. Costs for injectable forms cannot be reliably computed because dosage and frequency of injections are variable and must be individualized on the basis of disease severity and response of the patient.
9. Cost based on a person weighing 150 pounds (68 kilograms).

Brand Name/ Generic Name	Benefits and/ or Uses	Side Effects[1]

ASPIRIN OR ASPIRINLIKE ARTHRITIS DRUGS
continued

		breathing, mental confusion and fever, heart and breathing difficulties, and possible lowered resistance to bacteria and viruses.
Ecotrin **Esasprin** enteric-coated aspirin	Analgesic Anti-inflammatory	Causes fewer gastrointestinal problems than regular aspirin.
Trilisate choline magnesium trisalicylate	Anti-inflammatory Twice-a-day regimen Used for rheumatoid arthritis and osteoarthritis	Long term use or large doses may result in salicylate toxicity including vomiting, diarrhea, ulcer, ringing in the ears, loss of balance, headache, confusion, and drowsiness.

Interactions and Precautions[2]	Average Costs[3,4] (Drug, Lab, etc.)

Aspirin increases the excretion of the B vitamins in the urine.

Buffered aspirin may not provide protection from gastrointestinal problems.

Oral hyperglycemics are more effective when taken with salicylates.

Propranolol decreases aspirin's anti-inflammatory action.

Urinary alkalizers and phenobarbital each decrease the effectiveness of salicylates.

See also: Aspirin, all brands

Antacids will destroy the enteric coating while still in the stomach, increasing the risk of gastrointestinal problems.

$11.25–$16.88

More expensive than regular aspirin

Alcohol, corticosteroids, oxyphenbutazone, and phenylbutazone increase the risk of gastrointestinal ulcer.

Anticoagulants and oral hyperglycemics used with choline magnesium trisalicylate have an increased effect.

Antacids and urinary alkalizers decrease blood levels of choline magnesium trisalicylate which, in turn, decreases its effectiveness.

$58.03–$87.05

Brand Name/ Generic Name	Benefits and/ or Uses	Side Effects[1]

ASPIRIN OR ASPIRINLIKE ARTHRITIS DRUGS
continued

		Causes fewer gastrointestinal problems than aspirin.

Interactions and Precautions[2]	Average Costs[3],[4] (Drug, Lab, etc.)

Methotrexate blood levels become increased when taken with choline magnesium trisalicylate which, in turn, increases its toxic effects. Do not use together.

Probenecid and sulfinpyrazone effects are decreased when taken with choline magnesium trisalicylate.

Urinary acidifiers increase blood levels of choline magnesium trisalicylate which, in turn, increases its effectiveness.

Salicylates increase the rate of excretion of vitamin C in the urine which, in turn, decreases the excretion of aspirin, enhancing its activity.

Brand Name/ Generic Name	Benefits and/ or Uses	Side Effects[1]
ANALGESICS		
Datril **Excedrin** **Tylenol** acetaminophen (often in combination with aspirin)	Analgesic Used for osteoarthritis	Usually mild. May cause skin reactions. With high doses, vomiting, gastrointestinal hemorrhage, liver and kidney damage are possible. Use with caution with liver or kidney disorders. Long-term use may cause anemia and the formation of abnormal hemoglobin.
Empirin phenacetin or acetophenetidin (often in combination with aspirin, caffeine, or codeine)	Analgesic	May cause skin reactions, impaired thinking and concentration, anemia, and bone marrow depression. Long-term use may cause kidney damage and the formation of abnormal hemoglobin.

Interactions and Precautions[2]	Average Costs[3,4] (Drug, Lab, etc.)

Contains items that do not help relieve pain or inflammation.

Alcohol may enhance the activity of acetaminophen.

Barbiturates (including many sedatives) may reduce effectiveness of acetaminophen due to increased breakdown.

Acetaminophen alters the response to anticoagulant drugs and may increase the risk of abnormal bleeding.

$7.94–$15.87

Contains items that do not help relieve pain or inflammation.

Phenobarbital will hasten the elimination of phenacetin from the body and reduce its effectiveness.

$6.80

Brand Name/ Generic Name	Benefits and/ or Uses	Side Effects[1]

NONPRESCRIPTION TOPICAL ANALGESICS

**Absorbine Ar-
thritic**

Ben-Gay

Heet

Icy Hot

Mentholatum
 various ingre-
 dients, usually
 methyl salicy-
 late, menthol,
 and camphor

Counter-irritant
and mild local
anesthetic

Skin irritation
and blistering.

Interactions and Precautions[2]	Average Costs[3,4] (Drug, Lab, etc.)
Keep away from eyes and mucous membranes.	$3.39 per 3-ounce tube, used as needed for pain relief

Brand Name/ Generic Name	Benefits and/ or Uses	Side Effects[1]

NON-STEROIDAL ANTI-INFLAMMATORY (NSAI) DRUGS

Brand Name/ Generic Name	Benefits and/ or Uses	Side Effects[1]

Azolid
Butazolidin
Butazolidin Alka
  phenylbuta-
  zone
	Analgesic
	Anti-inflam-
	matory
	Used for rheu-
	matoid arthritis,
	bursitis, os-
	teoarthritis, an-
	kylosing
	spondylitis, and
	acute gout
		Nausea, jaundice,
		blurred vision,
		heartburn, indi-
		gestion, vomiting,
		red-violet rash
		characterized by
		target-shaped
		sores, diarrhea,
		and sores on the
		mucous mem-
		branes of the
		throat, skin, and
		gastrointestinal
		tract are possi-
		ble.
		
		May cause fluid
		retention,[5] eye
		problems, and
		gastrointestinal
		ulcer.
		
		Long-term use
		may cause thy-
		roid gland en-
		largements or
		blood disorders
		such as aplastic
		anemia due to
		bone marrow de-
		pression.

Interactions and Precautions[2]	Average Costs[3],[4] (Drug, Lab, etc.)

Valuable for short-term use only, due to potential toxicity.

Tartrazine (FD&C Yellow No. 5) used with phenylbutazone may cause allergic respiratory reactions.

Causes reduced iodine uptake and possible inhibition of thyroid activity.

Alcohol and anti-inflammatory drugs used with phenylbutazone increase the risk of gastrointestinal ulcer.

Antihistamines, barbiturates, digitoxin, griseofulvin, oral contraceptives, and zoxazolamine have decreased effects when used with phenylbutazone.

Hypoglycemia may be enhanced when phenylbutazone is used with antidiabetic drugs and insulin.

Coumarin anticoagulants taken with phenylbutazone may cause bleeding. Do not use together.

Aspirin, barbiturates, and some antidepressants reduce the effects of phenylbutazone.

Chloroquine and hydroxychloroquine taken with phenylbutazone cause increased sensitivity to the sun, resulting in skin rashes. Do not use together.

Phenytoin and lithium blood levels become increased when taken with

Gout: $4.99–$5.84 for 4-day treatment

Other arthritis: $5.36–$25.02[6]

Plus cost of periodic tests:

Complete blood cell counts

Upper gastrointestinal tests

Brand Name/ Generic Name	Benefits and/ or Uses	Side Effects[1]

NON-STEROIDAL ANTI-INFLAMMATORY (NSAI) DRUGS
continued

Clinoril sulindac	Anti-inflammatory Used for all major forms of arthritis including gout and painful shoulder	The most common effects are diarrhea or constipation, abdominal pain, nausea, and less frequently, ulceration and consequent blood loss, skin rash and itching, dizziness, and headache. Less common effects are vomiting and gas. Prolonged bleeding time, eye damage, and fluid retention[5] are possible.

Interactions and Precautions[2]	Average Costs[3,4] (Drug, Lab, etc.)

phenylbutazone which, in turn, increases their toxic effects.

Penicillin and sulfa drugs have increased effects when used with phenylbutazone.

Aspirin decreases blood levels of sulindac. Do not use together.	$20.30–$27.06 Plus cost of periodic eye examinations
Probenecid increases blood levels of sulindac which, in turn, decreases the uricosuric effect of probenecid.	
Other anti-inflammatory drugs used with sulindac will increase the risk of gastrointestinal ulcer.	

Brand Name/ Generic Name	Benefits and/ or Uses	Side Effects[1]

NON-STEROIDAL ANTI-INFLAMMATORY (NSAI) DRUGS
continued

Dolobid diflunisal	Analgesic Anti-inflammatory Twice-a-day regimen Used for osteoarthritis	The most common side effects are nausea, gastrointestinal pain, diarrhea, rash, and headache. Less common effects are vomiting, constipation, gas, sleepiness, insomnia, and dizziness. Prolonged bleeding time, eye damage, and fluid retention[5] are possible.
Feldene piroxicam	Analgesic Anti-inflammatory Once-a-day regimen Used for osteoarthritis and rheumatoid arthritis	Long-term use may result in blood disorders such as aplastic anemia, eye problems, kidney problems, and fluid retention.[5] Causes fewer gastrointestinal problems than aspirin but heartburn, nausea, and ulcers are still probable.

Interactions and Precautions[2]	Average Costs[3,4] (Drug, Lab, etc.)

Antacids reduce the blood level of diflunisal which, in turn, decreases its effectiveness.

Diflunisal increases blood clotting time, which interferes with the effects of anticoagulants.

Blood levels of some other anti-inflammatory drugs taken with diflunisal are reduced which, in turn, decreases their effectiveness.

$8.94–17.88

Plus cost of periodic eye examinations

Coumarin anticoagulants become less effective when taken with piroxicam.

Aspirin reduces blood levels of piroxicam which, in turn, reduces its effectiveness.

$34.80

Plus cost of periodic tests:

Complete blood cell counts

Eye examinations

Brand Name/ Generic Name	Benefits and/ or Uses	Side Effects[1]

NON-STEROIDAL ANTI-INFLAMMATORY (NSAI) DRUGS
continued

Brand Name/ Generic Name	Benefits and/ or Uses	Side Effects[1]
Indocin indomethacin	Analgesic Anti-inflam- matory Used for rheu- matoid arthritis, osteoarthritis, and ankylosing spondylitis	May cause head- ache, dizziness, loss of appetite, abdominal pain, nausea, vomiting, heartburn, diar- rhea, gastroin- testinal ulceration, con- stipation, tempo- rary loss of hair, and decreased resistance to in- fection. Blurring of vi- sion; gastroin- testinal bleeding; bone marrow de- pression; hepatitis; jaun- dice; and tingling, pain, numbness, and weakness in the hands or feet are possible.

Interactions and Precautions[2]	Average Costs[3,4] (Drug, Lab, etc.)

Indomethacin will mask the signs of infection. See your doctor if you suspect an infection.

Probenecid delays the excretion of indomethacin in the urine which, in turn, increases the effectiveness of indomethacin.

Aspirin, corticosteroids, and phenylbutazone each taken with indomethacin can increase the risk of gastrointestinal ulcer.

Coumarin anticoagulants taken with indomethacin may cause bleeding. Do not use together.

Thyroid medication effects on the heart and circulation become more probable and more risky.

Aspirin interferes with the uptake of indomethacin in the intestine.

Gout: $33.44

Other arthritis: $10.91–$32.72[6]

Plus cost of periodic tests:

Complete blood cell counts

Eye examinations

Liver function tests

Urinalysis

Brand Name/ Generic Name	Benefits and/ or Uses	Side Effects[1]

NON-STEROIDAL ANTI-INFLAMMATORY (NSAI) DRUGS
continued

Brand Name/ Generic Name	Benefits and/ or Uses	Side Effects[1]
Meclomen meclofenamate	Analgesic Anti-inflammatory Used for osteoarthritis and rheumatoid arthritis	Not recommended for initial use due to severe gastrointestinal effects such as diarrhea, nausea with or without vomiting, abdominal pain, gas, heartburn, and ulcers. Headache, dizziness, and skin rash are possible. May cause blood disorders such as decreased hemoglobin and hematocrit levels, and low white-cell counts which may call for discontinuation of drug use.

Interactions and Precautions[2]	Average Costs[3,4] (Drug, Lab, etc.)
Food has no effect on the absorption or effectiveness of meclofenamate. Take with food to relieve gastrointestinal problems.	$18.06–$36.12
	Plus cost of periodic tests:
Coumarin anticoagulants become more effective when taken with meclofenamate, which may cause bleeding.	Complete blood cell counts
	Eye examinations
Aspirin decreases blood levels of meclofenamate. Their use together causes more fecal blood loss than either drug used alone.	Hematocrit and hemoglobin level tests

Brand Name/ Generic Name	Benefits and/ or Uses	Side Effects[1]

NON-STEROIDAL ANTI-INFLAMMATORY (NSAI) DRUGS
continued

Motrin ibuprofen	Analgesic Anti-inflammatory Used for osteoarthritis and rheumatoid arthritis	Nausea, heartburn, abdominal pain, hair loss, dizziness, skin rash, gastrointestinal ulcer, fluid retention,[5] eye problems, and prolonged bleeding time are possible.
Nalfon fenoprofen	Analgesic Anti-inflammatory Used for osteoarthritis and rheumatoid arthritis	Nausea, indigestion, heartburn, sleepiness, dizziness, muscle weakness, skin rash and itching, heart palpitations, and nervousness. May make hearing problems worse in persons with impaired hearing, or cause ringing in the ears. May cause liver problems, eye problems, fluid

Interactions and Precautions[2]	Average Costs[3,4] (Drug, Lab, etc.)
Coumarin used with ibuprofen may cause bleeding. Do not use together. Aspirin reduces the anti-inflammatory activity of ibuprofen. Ibuprofen will mask the signs of infection. Contact your physician if you suspect an infection.	$21.56–$43.11 Plus cost of periodic tests: Complete blood cell counts Eye examinations Liver function tests
Food decreases fenoprofen blood levels. Therefore, take it 30 minutes before or 2 hours after meals.	$19.65–$39.30 Plus cost of periodic tests: Eye examinations Hearing tests Hemoglobin level tests Liver function tests

Brand Name/ Generic Name	Benefits and/ or Uses	Side Effects[1]

NON-STEROIDAL ANTI-INFLAMMATORY (NSAI) DRUGS
continued

		retention,[5] prolonged bleeding time, and gastrointestinal ulcer.
Naprosyn naproxen	Analgesic Anti-inflammatory Two- or three-times-a-day regimen Used for osteoarthritis, rheumatoid arthritis, and ankylosing spondylitis	Nausea, heartburn, abdominal pain, vomiting, gastrointestinal bleeding, headache, drowsiness, loss of balance, inability to concentrate, and depression are possible. May cause fluid retention,[5] eye problems, gastrointestinal ulcer, liver problems, and prolonged bleeding time.

Interactions and Precautions[2]	Average Costs[3,4] (Drug, Lab, etc.)
Aspirin increases the excretion of naproxen which, in turn, decreases its effects. Naproxen increases the effectiveness of some anticoagulants and antidiabetic drugs, phenytoin, and sulfonamides.	$19.43 Plus cost of periodic tests: Complete blood cell counts Eye examinations Hearing tests Hemoglobin level tests Kidney function tests Liver function tests

Brand Name/ Generic Name	Benefits and/ or Uses	Side Effects[1]

NON-STEROIDAL ANTI-INFLAMMATORY (NSAI) DRUGS
continued

| **Tandearil**
  oxyphen-
  butazone | Analgesic
Anti-inflam-
matory
Uricosuric
Used for rheu-
matoid arthritis,
acute gout, acute
osteoarthritis,
and ankylosing
spondylitis | Some gastroin-
testinal upset
such as nausea
and heartburn
are possible but
oxyphenbutazone
is less likely to
cause stomach
upset than phen-
ylbutazone.

Blood disorders
such as aplastic
anemia are possi-
ble.

May cause fluid
retention,[5] eye
problems, and
gastrointestinal
ulcer. |

Interactions and Precautions[2]	Average Costs[3,4] (Drug, Lab, etc.)

Valuable for short-term use only due to potential toxicity.	Gout: $8.44 for a 7-day treatment
Causes reduced iodine uptake and possible inhibition of thyroid activity.	Other arthritis: $22.02[6]
Alcohol and anti-inflammatory drugs used with oxyphenbutazone will increase the risk of gastrointestinal ulcer.	Plus cost of periodic tests:
Digitoxin has decreased effects when used with oxyphenbutazone.	Complete blood cell counts
Heparin used with oxyphenbutazone increases the risk of hemorrhage.	Eye examinations
Amodiaquine, chloroquine, gold salts, and hydroxychloroquine used with oxyphenbutazone increase the risk of skin rash.	
Hypoglycemia may be enhanced when oxyphenbutazone is used with insulin.	
Sulfonylureas and sulfonamides have increased effects when used with oxyphenbutazone.	
Phenytoin blood levels become increased when taken with oxyphenbutazone which, in turn, increases their effects.	
Coumarin anticoagulants may cause bleeding. Do not use together.	

Brand Name/ Generic Name	Benefits and/ or Uses	Side Effects[1]

NON-STEROIDAL ANTI-INFLAMMATORY (NSAI) DRUGS
continued

Brand Name/ Generic Name	Benefits and/ or Uses	Side Effects[1]
Tolectin **Tolectin DS** tolmetin	Analgesic Anti-inflammatory Used for juvenile rheumatoid arthritis, rheumatoid arthritis, and osteoarthritis	May cause gastrointestinal bleeding and ulcers. Nausea, abdominal pain, heartburn, gas, diarrhea, vomiting, headache, fluid retention,[5] dizziness, visual problems, and prolonged bleeding time are possible.
Zomax zomepirac	Analgesic Anti-inflammatory Used for osteoarthritis	Nausea, skin rash, drowsiness, muscle weakness, fluid retention,[5] elevated blood pressure, vomiting, indigestion, abdominal pain, excessive gas, diarrhea, constipation, and heartburn are possible. Long-term use may cause ul-

Interactions and Precautions[2]	Average Costs[3,4] (Drug, Lab, etc.)

Alcohol increases the risk of gastroin-testinal ulcer.

Anticoagulant drugs taken with tolmetin increase bleeding time. Do not use together.

Aspirin and aspirin-containing compounds decrease the effects of tolmetin. Do not use together.

Sodium bicarbonate increases the excretion of tolmetin which, in turn, decreases its effectiveness.

$35.01[6,7]

Plus cost of periodic tests:

Complete blood cell counts

Eye examinations

Kidney function tests

Liver function tests

Iron supplies may be depleted with long-term use. An iron supplement may be necessary.

Anticoagulants used with zomepirac are more effective, which results in increased bleeding time.

Zomepirac will mask the signs of infection. Contact your physician if you suspect an infection.

Food decreases the absorption of zomepirac.

Aspirin decreases blood levels of zomepirac which, in turn, reduces its effectiveness. Do not use together.

$38.52

Plus cost of periodic tests:

Complete blood cell counts

Eye examinations

Kidney function tests

Liver function tests

Urinalysis

Brand Name/ Generic Name	Benefits and/ or Uses	Side Effects[1]

NON-STEROIDAL ANTI-INFLAMMATORY (NSAI DRUGS *continued*

		cers, fluid retention,[5] kidney and urinary tract problems, gastrointestinal ulcer, and eye problems.

CORTICOSTEROID DRUGS

Cortisone cortisone	Anti-inflammatory Used for rheumatoid arthritis, acute psoriatic arthritis, juvenile rheumatoid arthritis, ankylosing spondylitis, bursitis, tenosynovitis, acute gout, osteoarthritis, and systemic lupus erythematosus	Increased susceptibility to infection and decreased wound healing. Long-term use may cause increased appetite, the development of diabetes, stomach ulcers, increased fat deposits on face and body trunk, thinning of skin, easy bruising, hair growth on the faces of women, glaucoma, cataracts, retarded

Interactions and Precautions[2]	**Average Costs[3,4] (Drug, Lab, etc.)**

Use with other non-steroid anti-inflammatory drugs may cause a severe allergic reaction.

Long-term use suppresses the body's production of steroids by the adrenal glands, producing a state of functional dependency.	$16.58 (oral)[6, 8]
Do not discontinue this drug abruptly.	Plus cost of periodic tests:
Hampers response to stress and physical trauma.	Eye examinations
Do not have vaccinations while taking cortisone because of decreased resistance to infection.	Measurement of blood potassium, blood sugar, and blood pressure
High-protein diets may be necessary during long-term use.	Rate of growth (children)
Tobacco smoking increases the amount of naturally produced cortisone which, in turn, increases the risk of side effects related to corticosteroid use.	
Barbiturates and other sedatives used with corticosteroids may cause oversedation.	

Brand Name/ Generic Name	Benefits and/ or Uses	Side Effects[1]

CORTICOSTEROID DRUGS *continued*

		growth and development in children, loss of muscle tone, and loss of texture and strength of bones, leading to osteoporosis and brittle bones.
		Large doses can cause high blood pressure, water imbalances such as fluid retention,[5] and increased excretion of potassium and calcium.
		Psychological instability such as mood swings, personality changes, insomnia, euphoria, and even severe depression or psychosis are possible.
		Flushing.

Interactions and Precautions[2]	Average Costs[3,4] (Drug, Lab, etc.)

Cholinelike drugs, coumarin anti-coagulants, insulin, and oral antidiabetic drugs have decreased effects when used with corticosteroids.

Thiazide diuretic may cause excessive loss of potassium.

Atropine-like drugs and stimulant drugs may cause increased internal eye pressure and lead to glaucoma.

Indomethacin and aspirin may increase the effects of corticosteroids, leading to increased risk of gastrointestinal ulcers.

Barbiturates, phenytoin, antihistamines, chloral hydrate, glutethimide, phenylbutazone, and propranolol decrease the effectiveness of corticosteroids.

Digitalis toxicity is possible due to increased potassium excretion. Do not use digitalis with corticosteroids.

Should not be taken with stomach ulcer, osteoporosis, or mental disorders.

Caution with heart failure, diabetes, infectious diseases, kidney failure, and in the elderly.

Brand Name/ Generic Name	Benefits and/ or Uses	Side Effects[1]

CORTICOSTEROID DRUGS *continued*

Brand Name/ Generic Name	Benefits and/ or Uses	Side Effects[1]
Aristocort **Kenacort** triamcinolone	*See:* Cortisone	Weight loss and dizziness may occur. *See also:* Cortisone
Celestone **Celestone phosphate** **Celestone soluspan** Betamethasone	*See:* Cortisone	*See:* Cortisone
Hydrocortone **Cortef** **Solu-cortef** hydrocortisone **(cortisol)**	*See:* Cortisone	Increased sweating, increased appetite, and weight gain are possible. *See also:* Cortisone
Decadron dexamethasone	*See:* Cortisone	Increased appetite and weight gain are possible. *See also:* Cortisone

Interactions and Precautions[2]	Average Costs[3,4] (Drug, Lab, etc.)
See: Cortisone	$119.25[7] *See:* Cortisone
See: Cortisone	$77.52 (oral)[6,8] *See:* Cortisone
Estrogen and oral contraceptives increase the effects of hydrocortisone. Monitor closely for corticosteroid toxicity. *See also:* Cortisone	$89.70 (oral)[7,8] *See:* Cortisone
See: Cortisone	$30.72 (oral)[7,8] *See:* Cortisone

Brand Name/ Generic Name	Benefits and/ or Uses	Side Effects[1]

CORTICOSTEROID DRUGS *continued*

Brand Name/ Generic Name	Benefits and/ or Uses	Side Effects[1]
Delta-cortef **Hydeltra TBA** prednisolone	*See:* Cortisone	Increased sweating, increased appetite, and weight gain are possible. *See also:* Cortisone
Deltasone **Metacorten** prednisone	*See:* Cortisone	Increased sweating, increased appetite, and weight gain are possible. *See also:* Cortisone
Depo-medrol **Medrol** methylprednisolone	*See:* Cortisone	Skin rash. *See also:* Cortisone
Haldrone paramethasone acetate	Use only for acute bursitis; not effective for chronic bursitis *See also:* Cortisone	*See:* Cortisone

Interactions and Precautions[2]	Average Costs[3,4] (Drug, Lab, etc.)
See: Cortisone	$—[8] *See:* Cortisone
See: Cortisone	$5.37[7] *See:* Cortisone
See: Cortisone	$60.16 (oral)[7,8] *See:* Cortisone
See: Cortisone	$61.31 *See:* Cortisone

Brand Name/ Generic Name	Benefits and/ or Uses	Side Effects[1]

ANTIMALARIAL DRUGS

Aralen **Avloclor** **Resochin** chloroquine	Antimalarial Remission-induc- ing Used for rheu- matoid arthritis	Susceptibility to sunburn, visual disturbances, and muscle weakness, headache, hair loss, nausea, vomiting, diarrhea, abdominal cramps, skin eruptions characterized by itching and redness. More severe effects are psychotic episodes, convulsions, diminished blood pressure and cardiovascular collapse, EKG changes, double vision, and difficulty in focusing the eyes. Long-term use may lead to retinal or corneal changes which may not be reversible, defects of color vision, pigmentation, op-

Interactions and Precautions[2]	Average Costs[3,4] (Drug, Lab, etc.)

Do not operate vehicles or machinery because visual problems may occur.

Do not use with bone marrow depressants, hemolytic drugs, or gold salts, phenylbutazone, and other agents that cause drug sensitization. (There are too many drugs to list here. For more information, see *Hazards of Medication,* by Eric W. Martin, Ph.D.)

Triamcinolone and phenylbutazone taken with chloroquine may cause skin rash. Do not use either with chloroquine.

Antipsoriatics are less effective when taken with chloroquine and their use together may cause a severe attack of psoriasis.

MAO inhibitors taken with chloroquine increase the risk of chloroquine toxicity and retinal damage.

$12.45

Plus cost of periodic tests:

Ankle and knee reflex

Complete blood cell counts

Eye examinations

Brand Name/ Generic Name	Benefits and/ or Uses	Side Effects[1]

ANTIMALARIAL DRUGS *continued*

		tic nerve damage, field of vision defects, and blindness.

Plaquenil
  hydroxychloro-
  quine
	Antimalarial
	Used for rheumatoid arthritis and systemic lupus erythematosus
		See: Aralen, Avloclor, Resochin

Interactions and Precautions[2]	Average Costs[3,4] (Drug, Lab, etc.)

Do not use with gold salts, phenylbutazone, and other agents that cause drug sensitization. (There are too many drugs to list here. For more information, see *Hazards of Medication,* by Eric W. Martin, Ph.D.)

$8.55–$17.10[6]

Plus cost of periodic tests:

Ankle and knee reflex

Complete blood cell counts

Eye examinations

Brand Name/ Generic Name	Benefits and/ or Uses	Side Effects[1]

URICOSURIC AGENTS

| **Anturane** sulfinpyrazone | Uricosuric agent Used for chronic gout | Causes development of kidney stones composed of uric acid. This risk can be reduced by drinking 2–3 quarts of water daily. Stomach irritation, nausea, vomiting, abdominal pain, and bone marrow depression are possible. Long-term use increases the risk of kidney damage. |

Interactions and Precautions[2]	**Average Costs**[3,4] **(Drug, Lab, etc.)**

This drug is very toxic. Remain under close medical supervision.

Use only after an acute attack of gout has subsided.

Insulin, penicillin, sulfa drugs, and sulfonylurea hypoglycemic drugs become more effective when each is taken with sulfinpyrazone. Use with caution.

Aspirin decreases the effectiveness of sulfinpyrazone and may cause bleeding. Do not use together.

Initial use may cause an acute attack of gout. Dosage adjustment and blood uric acid level test are necessary.

Coffee, tea, and cola beverages decrease the effectiveness of sulfinpyrazone.

Oral anticoagulants taken with sulfinpyrazone increase the risk of abnormal bleeding and hemorrhage.

Oral contraceptives become less effective when taken with sulfinpyrazone, increasing the frequency of breakthrough bleeding.

Probenecid increases the effectiveness of sulfinpyrazone.

Sulfinpyrazone is structurally related to phenylbutazone and oxyphenbutazone. *See also:* Azolid, Butazolidin, and Butazolidin Alka; and Tandearil.

$18.45

Plus cost of periodic tests:

Blood uric acid level tests

Complete blood cell counts

Kidney function tests

Brand Name/ Generic Name	Benefits and/ or Uses	Side Effects[1]

URICOSURIC AGENTS *continued*

Brand Name/ Generic Name	Benefits and/ or Uses	Side Effects[1]

Benemid
ColBenemid
  probenecid
  (Editor's note:
  ColBenemid is
  a combination
  of colchicine
  and pro-
  benecid.)
	Uricosuric agent
	Used for chronic
	gout
		Causes develop-
		ment of kidney
		stones composed
		of uric acid. This
		risk can be re-
		duced by
		drinking 2–3
		quarts of water
		daily.
		Headache, nau-
		sea, vomiting,
		loss of appetite,
		urinary fre-
		quency, skin rash,
		itching, fever,
		sore gums, flush-
		ing, dizziness,
		and anemia are
		possible.

Interactions and Precautions[2]	Average Costs[3,4] (Drug, Lab, etc.)

Use only after an acute attack of gout has subsided.	$4.00[6]
Coffee, tea, and cola beverages decrease the effectiveness of probenecid.	Plus cost of periodic tests:
Acetohexamide used with probenecid may cause hypoglycemia, upsetting smooth control of diabetes.	Complete blood cell counts
Allopurinol, indomethacin, nitrofuran-toin, and sulfinpyrazone have increased effects when taken with probenecid.	Kidney function tests Liver function tests
Penicillin has a three- to five-fold in-crease in effectiveness.	
Oral anticoagulants taken with pro-benecid increase the risk of abnormal bleeding or hemorrhage.	
Ethacrynic acid has reduced diuretic effects when taken with probenecid.	
Para-aminosalicylic acid and sul-fonamide slow the excretion of probenecid and increase its blood levels.	
Aspirin, aspirinlike drugs, and eth-acrynic acid decrease the effectiveness of probenecid.	
Thiazide diuretics decrease the effec-tiveness of probenecid by increasing the level of uric acid in the blood.	

Brand Name/ Generic Name	Benefits and/ or Uses	Side Effects[1]

ANTIGOUT DRUGS

Brand Name/ Generic Name	Benefits and/ or Uses	Side Effects[1]
Colchicine **ColBenemid** colchicine (Editor's note: ColBenemid is a combination of colchicine and pro-benecid.)	Antigout agent Used for acute gout	Abdominal pain, nausea, vomiting, diarrhea, and blood disorders due to bone marrow depression are possible. Long-term use may result in numbness in hands and feet, loss of hair, inflammation of colon, liver damage, and aplastic anemia. Sperm production may be affected, possibly leading to birth defects if child is conceived while the father is taking colchicine.

Interactions and Precautions[2]	Average Costs[3,4] (Drug, Lab, etc.)

B_{12} is not absorbed well when taken with colchicine. B_{12} supplementation may be necessary.

Acidifying agents decrease the effectiveness of colchicine.

Alkalizing agents increase the effectiveness of colchicine.

Analgesics, narcotic drugs, sedatives, sleep-inducing drugs, and tranquilizers taken with colchicine may cause over-sedation.

Stimulants such as adrenaline, ephedrine, and epinephrine have increased effectiveness when taken with colchicine.

Anticoagulants and antihypertensives have decreased effectiveness when taken with colchicine.

Colchicine can lower body temperature and lead to hypothermia, especially in the elderly.

Acute gout attack: $2.30 for a 24-hour treatment

Chronic gout: $6.66–$8.66

Plus cost of periodic tests:

Blood uric acid level tests

Complete blood cell counts

Liver function tests

Sperm analysis

Brand Name/ Generic Name	Benefits and/ or Uses	Side Effects[1]

ANTIGOUT DRUGS *continued*

Brand Name/ Generic Name	Benefits and/ or Uses	Side Effects[1]
Zyloprim allopurinol	Antigout agent Used for chronic gout	An increase in the frequency and severity of acute gout may occur during the first several weeks of drug use. Skin rash, hives, itching, fever, nausea, vomiting, drowsiness, headache, dizziness, and loss of scalp hair are possible. Blood disorders due to bone marrow depression, hepatitis with or without jaundice, and kidney damage are possible.

Interactions and Precautions[2]	Average Costs[3,4] (Drug, Lab, etc.)
Coffee, tea, and cola beverages decrease the effectiveness of allopurinol.	$8.73
Drink no less than 2–3 quarts of liquid every 24 hours.	Plus cost of periodic tests:
Azathioprine and mercaptopurine have increased effectiveness when taken with allopurinol. Dosages may need to be reduced by one-third to one-quarter.	Complete blood cell counts
Oral anticoagulants taken with allopurinol may cause bleeding. Dosage adjustment may be necessary.	Eye examinations Kidney function tests
Iron may accumulate when taken with allopurinol. Do not use together.	Liver function tests
The action of theophylline is prolonged when taken with allopurinol.	
Acetohexamide and probenecid increase the effectiveness of allopurinol.	
Ethacrynic acid and thiazide diuretics decrease the effectiveness of allopurinol.	

Brand Name/ Generic Name	Benefits and/ or Uses	Side Effects[1]

GOLD SALTS AND PILLS

Myochrysine
  gold sodium
  thiomalate
	Anti-inflam-
	matory
	Remission-induc-
	ing
	Intermuscular in-
	jections
	Used for juvenile
	rheumatoid ar-
	thritis
		Joint pain some-
		times occurs
		following an in-
		jection, lasting for
		as long as a day
		or two after injec-
		tion.
		
		Flushing, fainting,
		dizziness, sweat-
		ing, nausea,
		vomiting, malaise,
		weakness, diar-
		rhea, abdominal
		cramps, colitis,
		and photosen-
		sitivity are
		possible.
		
		Gold agents ac-
		cumulate in the
		body and can
		cause toxic
		effects at any
		time during treat-
		ment.
		
		Kidney damage is
		common. There-
		fore, urinalysis is
		necessary before
		every injection. If
		excess protein or
		blood is found,
		the drug should

Interactions and Precautions[2]	Average Costs[3,4] (Drug, Lab, etc.)

Gold salts are last-resort drugs to be used when other anti-inflammatory drugs provide no relief.

Para-aminobenzoic acid aggravates the dermatitis and fever associated with gold therapy.

Chloroquine taken with gold therapy increases the risk of gold toxicity.

Do not use with hydroxychloroquine, phenylbutazone, and other agents that cause drug sensitization and dermatitis. (There are too many drugs to list here. For more information, see *Hazards of Medication,* by Eric W. Martin, Ph.D.)

Corticosteroids decrease the effectiveness of gold therapy and increase the risk of gold toxicity.

Oxyphenbutazone and phenylbutazone increase the risk of gold toxicity and blood disorders.

Penicillamine and other immunosuppressive drugs increase the risk of gold toxicity. Do not use together.

$8.09

Plus cost of periodic tests:

Complete blood cell counts, platelet counts (before treatment and every 2 weeks afterwards)

Urinalysis (before treatment and before every injection)

Brand Name/ Generic Name	Benefits and/ or Uses	Side Effects[1]

GOLD SALTS AND PILLS *continued*

be discontinued.
The following side effects suggest the development of gold toxicity, and no further injections should be given until tests show some other cause for their presence:

blood disorders (fatal blood disorders may occur suddenly) and albumin in the urine, dermatitis, inflammation of the mucous membranes of the mouth, metallic taste, jaundice, pinpoint hemorrhages in the skin, and exfoliate dermatitis characterized by skin rash on

Interactions and
Precautions[2]

Average Costs[3,4]
(Drug, Lab, etc.)

Brand Name/ Generic Name	Benefits and/ or Uses	Side Effects[1]

GOLD SALTS AND PILLS *continued*

		the whole body, peeling, itching, and loss of hair.
Ridaura auranofin	Anti-inflammatory Remission-inducing Pill form Not yet approved in U.S. Intended for use in rheumatoid arthritis	Gastrointestinal upset and skin rash are possible. Complete information is not available but gold in pill form may produce fewer side effects than injected gold salts. *See also:* Myochrysine
Solganal gold thioglucose	Anti-inflammatory Remission-inducing Intermuscular injections Used for juvenile rheumatoid arthritis and rheumatoid arthritis	*See:* Myochrysine

Interactions and Precautions[2]	Average Costs[3,4] (Drug, Lab, etc.)

Information not available.

Information not available.

See: Myochrysine

$6.77

Brand Name/ Generic Name	Benefits and/ or Uses	Side Effects[1]

IMMUNOSUPPRESSIVE AND CYTOTOXIC DRUGS

Cytoxan

  cyclophospha-mide

Immunosuppressive

Currently being investigated for use in rheumatoid arthritis and systemic lupus erythematosus

Decreased resistance to infection and slow wound healing are possible.

Blood disorders are possible due to bone marrow depression. Therefore, frequent blood tests are necessary.

Loss of hair, skin rash, darkening of skin and fingernails, nausea, vomiting, loss of appetite, mouth ulcers, bloody diarrhea, fluid retention,[5] liver and kidney damage, severe inflammation of the bladder, reduced ovarian and testicular function, and cancer are possible.

Can cause significant

Interactions and Precautions[2]	Average Costs[3,4] (Drug, Lab, etc.)

Drink at least 2 quarts of water every 24 hours.

Oral antidiabetic drugs and insulin have increased effectiveness and may cause hypoglycemia.

Allopurinol taken with cyclophosphamide can cause bone marrow depression. Do not use together.

Anesthetics taken with cyclophosphamide can be fatal. Discontinue use at least 12 hours beforehand.

Barbiturates increase the effectiveness of cyclophosphamide.

Prednisolone decreases the effectiveness of cyclophosphamide.

$64.26 (oral)[7,8,9]

Plus cost of periodic tests:

Complete blood cell counts (initially these tests should be performed every 2–4 days)

Kidney function tests

Liver function

Thyroid function tests

Urinalysis

Brand Name/ Generic Name	Benefits and/ or Uses	Side Effects[1]

IMMUNOSUPPRESSIVE AND CYTOTOXIC DRUGS
continued

		chromosomal changes in the egg and sperm.
Imuran azathioprine	Anti-inflammatory Immunosuppressive Used for rheumatoid arthritis	Severe anemia due to bone marrow depression, and a reduction in the number of leukocytes and blood platelets may occur. These are serious blood disorders, therefore frequent blood tests are necessary. Serious infections and the development of cancer are constant hazards. Nausea and vomiting may occur within the first few months of treatment. Muscle wasting and skin rashes are possible.

Interactions and Precautions[2]	Average Costs[3,4] (Drug, Lab, etc.)

Azathioprine is a last-resort drug to be used when other anti-inflammatory drugs or gold drugs provide no relief.

Allopurinol interferes with the metabolism of azathioprine, increasing the risk of toxic effects. The dosage of azathioprine should be reduced by one-third to one-quarter of the usual dose.

Corticosteroids taken with azathioprine for long periods of time may cause negative nitrogen balance, muscle wasting, and malignancy.

$16.01–$32.03 (oral)[8,9]

Plus cost of periodic tests:

Complete blood cell counts, platelet counts (initially both these tests should be performed weekly)

Brand Name/ Generic Name	Benefits and/ or Uses	Side Effects[1]

IMMUNOSUPPRESSIVE AND CYTOTOXIC DRUGS
continued

Brand Name/ Generic Name	Benefits and/ or Uses	Side Effects[1]
Mexate methotrexate	Immunosuppressive Used for systemic lupus erythematosus	Gastrointestinal ulcers, loss of hair, skin rashes, and reduced ovarian and testicular function may occur. Kidney, liver, lung, and nerve damage is possible and may be fatal. Blood disorders such as a decreased number of leukocytes and blood platelets, nausea, vomiting, diarrhea, and decreased resistance to infection are possible.

Interactions and Precautions[2]	Average Costs[3,4] (Drug, Lab, etc.)
Para-aminobenzoic acid, chloramphenicol, phenytoin, salicylates, sulfonamides, tetracyclines, and thiazide diuretics increase the effectiveness of methotrexate which, in turn, increases the risk of toxicity.	$32.56 (oral)[7,8] Plus cost of periodic tests: Complete blood cell counts
Alcohol taken with methotrexate may cause cirrhosis of the liver, respiratory failure, and coma. Do not use together.	
Do not have vaccinations while taking methotrexate because of decreased resistance to infections.	
Mercaptopurine taken with methotrexate may cause blood disorders.	

Brand Name/ Generic Name	Benefits and/ or Uses	Side Effects[1]

REMISSION-INDUCING DRUGS

Cuprimine **Depen** penicillamine	Chelating agent Used for rheu- matoid arthritis	Loss of appetite, explosive vomit- ing, loss of taste, sores on mucous membranes, ex- cretion of protein in urine, bone marrow prob- lems, gastrointestinal problems, skin rashes, excessive skin wrinkling, and kidney prob- lems may occur.
		Use has resulted in fatalities due to aplastic anemia, blood disorders, kidney disease, and myasthenia gravis.
		Protein and blood in the urine are possible and may lead to kidney disease.
		Excessive cough- ing or wheezing may occur and suggest pulmo- nary problems.

Interactions and Precautions[2]	Average Costs[3,4] (Drug, Lab, etc.)

Due to excessive and severe side effects, use only when all other treatments fail. Remain under close medical supervision.

Food decreases the absorption of penicillamine. Take at least 1 hour before meals and at least 1 hour apart from any other drug, food, or milk.

Pyridoxine-dependent enzymes may be inhibited by penicillamine. A pyridoxine (B_6) supplement may be necessary.

Do not use with gold salts or antimalarials, cytotoxic drugs, oxyphenbutazone, or phenylbutazone because penicillamine increases the risk of toxicity.

Persons allergic to penicillin may also be sensitive to penicillamine.

Mineral supplements may block the activity of penicillamine.

Gout: $103.20

Other arthritis: $6.45–$12.90[6]

Plus cost of periodic tests:

Liver function tests

White and differential blood cell counts, direct platelet counts, and hemoglobin level tests every 2 weeks for the first 6 months of treatment

Brand Name/ Generic Name	Benefits and/ or Uses	Side Effects[1]

REMISSION-INDUCING DRUGS *continued*

| | | Fever in the second and third week accompanied by skin rash is serious and the drug should be discontinued and another alternative tried. |
| | | Lupuslike syndrome may develop with or without the blood complications. |

Interactions and Precautions[2]	Average Costs[3,4] (Drug, Lab, etc.)

Brand Name/ Generic Name	Benefits and/ or Uses	Side Effects[1]

MISCELLANEOUS DRUGS

Brand Name/ Generic Name	Benefits and/ or Uses	Side Effects[1]
Ketrax **Solaskil** levamisole	Nematocidal agent Not approved for use in U.S.	May cause nausea and vomiting, abdominal discomfort, headaches, dizziness, hypotension, and a decreased number of white blood cells.
(None) orgotein	Anti-inflammatory Remission-inducing Not approved for use in U.S. Intended for use for osteoarthritis and rheumatoid arthritis.	Local pain following injection into joint. This drug is still under investigation.

Interactions and Precautions[2]	Average Costs[3,4] (Drug, Lab, etc.)
Information not available.	Information not available.
Information not available.	Information not available.

Index

Page numbers in **boldface** type indicate tables.

More Fine Health Related Books You Will Want